P9-CJC-615

TOP TIPS
for Girls ·

REAL ADVICE
FROM REAL WOMEN
FOR REAL LIFE

TOP TIPS
for Girls

REAL ADVICE
FROM REAL WOMEN
FOR REAL LIFE

Kate Reardon

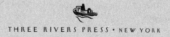

THREE RIVERS PRESS · NEW YORK

For my family

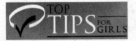

Copyright © 2008 by Top Tips Ltd.

All rights reserved.
Published in the United States by Three Rivers Press, an imprint
of the Crown Publishing Group, a division of Random House, Inc.,
New York.
www.crownpublishing.com

Three Rivers Press and the Tugboat design are registered trademarks
of Random House, Inc.

All tips originally appeared online at www.toptips.com. Originally
published in book form in Great Britain by Headline Publishing
Group, London.

Library of Congress Cataloging-in-Publication Data
Reardon, Kate.
   Top tips for girls : real advice from real women for real life /
Kate Reardon.—1st ed.
     Includes index.
     1. Women—Conduct of life.   2. Girls—Conduct of life.   I. Title.
     BJ1610.R43 2008
     646.700835'2—dc22   2008006866
     ISBN 978-0-307-40669-9

Printed in the United States of America

Design by Nora Rosansky

10 9 8 7 6 5 4 3 2 1

First American Edition

CONTENTS

INTRODUCTION

WHEN my brother and I were little and complained of sore throats, my mother would make us sleep wearing her infamous lard-and-nutmeg plaster around our necks. It was a piece of cotton (usually ripped from an old T-shirt) three or four inches wide, spread with lard and sprinkled with ground nutmeg. Yes, it was disgusting, but more annoyingly, it actually worked. She maintains that it's an old Victorian remedy, told to her by her mother and used as far back as her grandmother's own childhood in 1870.

This is what *Top Tips for Girls* is all about—not necessarily torture of small children with animal by-products, but about collecting all those little tips and tricks that get us through life. Whether these helpful hints have been passed down the generations or we figure them out for ourselves, every woman has her own arsenal of them.

In the past we inherited our grandmothers' cookbooks, and our mothers, sisters, and aunts would pass on their own hard-won wisdom. But previous generations' abandonment of traditional roles, combined with the breakdown of the extended family, means that we now rely on our friends and peers, who have as little life experience as we do. It isn't surprising that many modern women are feeling ill equipped and isolated. In the absence of the traditional network of support, each time we spill red wine on the carpet, can't get our kids to sleep, or have a disastrous encounter with hair dye, we have to reinvent the wheel.

Now that the family-authored encyclopedia are no longer within reach, and if our friends are as clueless as we are, we rather desperately seek guidance from celebrity lifestyle gurus. The success of these replacement grandmothers is testament to our need for advice on matters of the home, hearth, and heart. But many of these chic and fabulous guides are dictatorial, patronizing, or authored by people who can't remember the last time they did their own laundry. And so often they are delivered in a twinkly, cutesy style that demeans our search for knowledge and assistance. This is real life, not some fey 1950s muffin-baking championship.

So to create the ultimate compendium of real women's wisdom and advice, I started the website toptipsforgirls .com. Out of the gate, I want to make it clear that I am not the guru. I am as, if not more, clueless than the next woman who failed to listen to her mother. Displaying only user-generated content, the site is written by the women who visit it; none claims to be an expert, but some may share the best way to stop a toddler's tantrum and others may have discovered the all-time greatest exfoliation method. Harnessing the awesome power of pooled resources, toptipsforgirls.com has become a platform for women to share life-enhancing tips and tricks, combined with the remembered fragments of their grandmothers' wisdom.

With more than a million hits in the first month, the site was immediately a success. This is perhaps because women thrive in communities, and feeling the absence of traditional ones we are increasingly turning to Internet-based societies. Toptipsforgirls.com attracts women from twenty to eighty, the joy being that the youngsters can advise their elders on matters of fashion, beauty, and technology, while the older ones can share a lifetime's experience of love, cooking, and child care. Everyone has something to share, and what may be as plain as the nose on her face to one woman may be rocket science to another.

The website was also partly inspired by a childless woman of fifty who recently confided that although she has come to terms with never becoming a mother, what really upsets her is that she doesn't have anyone to pass her mother's fabulous chocolate cake recipe on to. Family recipes and the tricks we hand down through the generations are our DNA. Although seemingly frivolous, they are certainly more valuable and important than the color of our eyes, the curliness of our hair, and whether we are prone to double chins. Our urge to share our tips is about passing on that DNA. So our friends and acquaintances take the place of our mothers and daughters in this evolutionary chain of tips.

My great-aunt Lala married in her fifties and so remained childless. This made her the greatest aunt ever. When her young relatives visited, she would settle us in a great big armchair in front of the television, and we would only have to snap our imperious little fingers for her to happily bring us snacks and treats. But more important, she also took the greatest care to teach all the women in our family how to cook, sew, make things, and look after ourselves.

Some of her tips were a little odd, such as drinking a solution of baking soda to ward off colds in the belief that the fizz makes you burp out the germs. But Lala's DNA lives on, if only because I still know how to keep sewing thread from tangling (thread your needle before you cut the thread off the spool).

Even if we don't have children or no longer live across the road from our trusted female relatives, women have an intrinsic and irresistible urge to seek and give advice (unlike many men, who appear happy to drive twenty miles in the wrong direction, literally or emotionally, because they don't want to ask for help). It is part of the way in which we communicate with one another. While men can walk into a roomful of strangers and bond over the big game, women who have only just met can instantly and unthreateningly connect via the universal language of beauty tips.

This book is a compilation of the best tips from toptips forgirls.com. It has been written by a community of your sisters from Honolulu to Beijing who have little in common other than access to a computer and knowing what it's like to battle unruly hair. They have all been generous enough to share what works for them, and for that I thank them wholeheartedly.

The tips you'll find run the gamut from the straightforwardly practical, such as "How to remove fake tan streaks," to the more poignant, such as "How to cope with bereavement." Some may seem pretty weird but are worth a try—who knew that you could iron your clothes using hair flat irons? And, as in life, sometimes there are multiple solutions for one problem, as with How to get over him and How to be happy.

As one wise tipster said, "We're here for a good time, not for a long time." So don't learn everything the hard way; listen to the women who have been there, done that, and gotten the red-wine stain out of the rug.

The tips in this book are the opinions of people who have contributed to my website. I haven't rigorously tested them all; they simply sounded like they made good sense, and my guess is, most of them will work. So if you make holes in your sweaters, turn your eyebrows green, or your family disowns you because you followed any of the tips in this book, it's not my fault. (And if you choose to smear yourself with lard and nutmeg, my mother would probably like to hear from you.)

If you've got a better idea for any of the tips you find in this book, or tips not found here, do please go to www.toptipsforgirls.com and let us all know.

· HOME ·

or, Martha Stewart, eat your heart out.

Just imagine, if you had absolutely nothing else to do at all, how magnificent your home would look. I'm thinking fresh flowers, bread baking in a spotless oven, no piles of laundry, perhaps a filing system for socks. Yup, we'd all be five-star generals of the home—if only we didn't have jobs, and children, and a life. Modern woman is cursed by unrealistic expectations; just as she is expected to snap back into a girlish figure moments after childbirth, her home is now also supposed to be effortlessly perfect. The home is becoming an ever-more competitive arena. Women who once competed for the attentions of alpha (or perhaps beta) males can now devote years of experience and cunning to outdoing one another on the domestic front. For an unfair advantage, read the following.

HOW TO GET RID OF HOUSEFLIES

Put some eucalyptus oil on a cloth, open the door wide, and wave the cloth vigorously, working toward the door. Flies will rapidly disappear.

—*Caroline*

HOW TO GET RID OF ANTS

Ants pretty much steer clear of anything that is "powdery," so to speak. I believe it has to do with the fact that any powder disrupts their senses and makes their little legs not able to, say, climb a wall; they just fall right off. I've had really good luck with using baby powder.

—*lisaveronica*

HOW TO CLEAN WINDOWS AND SHINY METAL WITHOUT CHEMICALS

For floors and counters, use 1 part vinegar and 3 parts water. For glass, use 1 part vodka, 1 part grapefruit juice, and 6 parts water.

—*Amy*

HOW TO CLEAN WINDOWS

Add dishwasher rinse aid to your bucket of water instead of soap.

—*Moodykat*

HOW TO REMOVE STICKY TAPE FROM GLASS

Put some nail-polish remover on a bit of cotton and rub away.

—*buckridge*

HOW TO MAKE A CANDLE FIT
A TOO-SMALL CANDLESTICK

Hold the end in very hot water and it will become soft enough to be jammed in tight.

—*Tawny*

HOW TO KEEP CANDLES BURNING LONGER

Store them in the freezer—this will add hours of additional burn time.

—*Estelle*

HOW TO GET CANDLE WAX OFF
WOOD FURNITURE OR CARPET

Get a large brown envelope or a paper grocery bag and a hot iron. Place the brown envelope over the wax stain, then press the hot iron on top of the envelope. The iron heats up the candle wax and the brown paper absorbs the hot wax, thus removing it from the carpet or furniture.

—*lulu8749*

HOW TO BUILD A GREAT FIRE

If you want big flames, build a tepee shape with your logs against the back of the fireplace.

—*Belinda*

HOW TO STOP A FIRE FROM SMOKING UP A ROOM

Roll up a few sheets of newspaper, light them, and hold them up the chimney before you light the fire. This will heat the chimney and create a draft that will suck the smoke upward. And don't forget to have your chimney swept regularly.

—*Melanie*

HOW TO SAVE THE FLATTENED CARPET UNDERNEATH YOUR FURNITURE

Place a damp towel over the area and iron it. The steam will restore the carpet's natural fluff.

—*Chelsea*

Leave a small ice cube in the indent. Once it melts and dries a bit, vacuum with the brush attachment.

—*JCF*

HOW TO CLEAN LAMP SHADES

I keep a soft-bristled paintbrush around for this sort of task. It helps remove dust in tight ridges and grooves. I also use it for dusting bookcases and electronic equipment. These brushes are inexpensive and can be rinsed out.

—*melaniezelanie*

HOW TO CHANGE A DUVET COVER EASILY

If you can drop both duvet and cover, holding the corners, over a stairwell and shake, this should work well. (Try storing linen inside one of the set's pillowcases; it saves a lot of time searching for a matching set when changing the bed.)

—*josie*

HOW TO DOWNSIZE TO A SMALLER KITCHEN

Instead of putting all utensils, cutlery, plates, and glasses away in their usual place, put them in a separate box or tub each time you finish using them. Within a few weeks, you will see exactly what you actually use, rather than all that junk that's just filling up your kitchen.

—*Helen*

HOW TO HAVE A TIDY HOUSE WITH NO EFFORT

Instead of sitting gazing moronically at dumb ads on TV, get up and do something useful during every commercial break. That way, tidying, cleaning a sink, sorting laundry, going through paperwork, or washing the dishes gets done in short bursts without becoming a major task.

—*aitch*

Each day, set an egg timer for fifteen minutes and get as *much* done as you can in that time. Sadly, I get extra excited when I finish and realize I've done more than the day before. Ah, the satisfaction.

—*CassandraM*

HOW TO GET GREASE AND FINGERPRINTS OFF THE WALLS

Use a slice of white bread to rub off any dirt or stains.

—*yvonne1987*

HOW TO STOP CHILDREN'S JUNK FROM
TAKING OVER THE WHOLE HOUSE

Let each child choose his or her own big box (mine chose a large, brightly colored plastic one) and a smaller one. At the end of the day, have "tidy up time" and give a treat to the tidiest (my kids chose extra time in the bath or extra bubbles . . . they're teenagers now, so those treats seem very tame!). All the toys go into the big box; the smaller box holds crayons or "losable" things. Then there is only one box to put away in the bedroom (or hide behind the sofa if mother-in-law is on the horizon).

—faylin4

HOW TO MAKE ALMOST ANY ABHORRENT
TASK GO FASTER

Set a timer for thirty minutes and do nothing but that task while the timer is on. When the timer goes off, give yourself permission to be done. You've been productive and now you can take a break. I find this makes a big difference and helps me get done those tasks I don't particularly enjoy.

—CeeVee

HOW TO PUT AWAY LAUNDRY

Always put fresh laundry *under* the pile of similar things, or at the farther reaches of your closet. That way you'll actually wear all your T-shirts and underwear, instead of the same three over and over again.

—Tawny

HOW TO STOP STATIC FROM BUILDING UP FROM THE DRYER

Pour a bit of laundry softener onto an old washcloth and put it in with your drying.

—*Brianne*

HOW TO HANG SWEATERS ON A CLOTHESLINE

Take an old pair of hose and thread the legs through the arms of your sweater so that the waist is sticking out through the neck. Then you can clip the feet and waistband of the tights to the line—it stops those annoying clothespin marks on your sweaters.

—*Margot*

HOW TO GET CHEWING GUM OUT OF FABRICS

If the gum is embedded, rub with vinegar (preferably white), and the gum will break up and fall away.

—*Caprice*

HOW TO REMOVE WATERMARKS ON DARK WOOD

This is a really yucky solution, but it does work: If you have white watermarks on mahogany or dark polished wood, mix a paste of olive oil and cigarette ash and work it into the mark. It will come out, and the smell will disappear quite quickly!

—*Sage*

It sounds pretty daunting, but metal polish does work. Put a little bit on a soft cloth and work it in over the watermark, then polish off with another clean, soft cloth.

—*loops*

HOW TO PROTECT WALLS FROM BEING
MARKED BY THE TOPS OF LADDERS

Put old socks over the tops of stepladders so that they don't mark walls when they're leaned against them.

—*Georgia*

HOW TO HANG WALLPAPER

Hanging wallpaper is easier if you put the paste on the wall rather than on the wallpaper first.

—*Scout*

HOW TO FILL TINY CRACKS WHEN
PAINTING WOODWORK

Add a bit of flour to your paint.

—*Fern*

HOW TO ELIMINATE PAINT SMELLS
WHEN DECORATING

Before painting, add a few drops of vanilla extract to the paint and mix it in well. If you're using white paint, make sure you get clear vanilla extract.

—*lnmop*

HOW TO MAKE A ROOM SMELL NICE

Place a dryer sheet used in tumble dryers on the top of a radiator. When the radiator is on, the sheet warms up and the smell fills the room.

—*BarbaraClark*

HOW TO CLEAN DECANTERS AND ODD-SHAPED VASES

To clean decanters, fill a quarter of the way up with warm water, add crushed eggshell, and shake.

—*Scout*

Denture-cleaner tabs are effective, as is a small amount of washing powder or dishwasher powder—just make sure the decanter is well rinsed afterward. (Because we don't drink whiskey, we didn't know that the expensive whiskey in the decanter we had "cleaned" tasted soapy!)

—*charpur*

HOW TO CLEAN ANTIQUE IVORY PIANO KEYS

I heard that toothpaste is good on white piano keys. It makes sense, because tusks are elephant's teeth after all.

—*ValW*

HOW TO REMOVE SCUFF MARKS FROM LINOLEUM FLOORS

Use WD40 to remove marks left by shoes and sneakers.

—*jackandclaire*

HOW TO KEEP SILVER CLEAN

If you keep a stick of chalk in with your silver jewelry, it keeps the jewelry from tarnishing—it is also great for silver dinner services. My grandmother taught me this and it does work.

—*diamondsparkle*

HOW TO CLEAN SILVER

Line the bottom of a large bowl (or the sink) with aluminum foil.
Fill it with hot, hot water, add baking soda, and put in your silver
pieces. The tarnish will come off the silver and stick to the aluminum foil all by itself—no need to scrub or anything. Works
like a charm in just a couple of minutes.

—*lalaland*

HOW TO REMOVE RUST MARKS FROM CHROME

Scrunch up some aluminium foil and rub away the rust—I tried
it and it really worked.

—*animal2415*

HOW TO STOP A DOOR FROM SQUEAKING

If you don't have any oil or are worried about getting a mess on
your carpet, try a tiny blob of washing-up liquid on the hinges. It
sounds mad, but my grandmother has sworn by it for years.

—*saz57*

HOW TO REMOVE A BROKEN LIGHTBULB

Take half an uncooked potato (the big, starchy kind) and stick it
over the ragged lightbulb end to protect you from broken glass.
Twist the lightbulb out of the socket.

—*rsjdooley*

HOW TO STOP CURTAIN TRACKS FROM STICKING

If your curtains don't run smoothly on the curtain track, wipe
the track with a little furniture polish. It works wonders.

—*Rosbod*

HOW TO CLEAN LEATHER FURNITURE

If you are out of leather cleaner, a baby wipe is excellent; if it's good enough for babies' bottoms, it's good enough for leather.

—*housewifeandsuperstar*

HOW TO STOP FLOORBOARDS FROM CREAKING

If you dust talcum powder between the floorboards, it sometimes stops them from creaking.

—*Samantha*

HOW TO MAKE DRAWERS RUN MORE SMOOTHLY

If old wooden drawers are sticking, try rubbing the edges with old candles.

—*Bridget*

HOW TO PICK UP BROKEN GLASS

Use a wet cotton ball; it should pick up even the tiny shards.

—*Noelle*

Use a slice of fresh bread; it easily picks up the smallest bits of broken glass.

—*Scarlett*

Think there are still shards of glass that you might have missed? Shine a flashlight over the area. Any remaining glass should shimmer in the light.

—*Holly*

HOW TO REMOVE PAINT FROM SKIN

For a nonirritating paint remover, use cooking oil.

   —*Lara*

HOW TO FIX SCREWS IN AWKWARD PLACES

Use Blu Tack to stick the screw head to the screwdriver. This is brilliant in cases when gravity is against you, for example, if the screw has to go in upside down.

   —*LevantineLass*

HOW TO REMOVE SOAP SCUM FROM CHILDREN'S BATH TOYS OR KEEP IT FROM BUILDING UP

Run them through the dishwasher.

   —*sk1970*

HOW TO CLEAN HARD-WATER STAINS FROM GLASS SHOWER DOORS

I use lemon juice—the acid dissolves the lime scale. I also use a squeegee (used when washing and drying windows) to wipe the glass right after showering to remove excess water.

   —*star*

HOW TO CLEAN TAPS

Keep an old toothbrush with your cleaning kit; every time you clean the basin or the sink, use it to scrub around the base of the tap—much easier than trying to get a cloth in there, and it keeps the lime scale down.

   —*Labink*

Soak a piece of paper towel in white vinegar and wrap it around the base of the tap. Leave it for as long as possible—at least half an hour. Gets rid of lime scale like a dream.

—*karenannerichards*

HOW TO TEMPORARILY STOP THE ANNOYING NOISE OF A DRIP FROM A LEAKING TAP

Tie dental floss around the bottom of the tap and let the floss tail hang into the bowl of the sink. Water will travel down the floss into the basin rather than dropping from the tap.

—*Tonya*

HOW TO WASH GLASSES

Remember when hand washing glasses that it's the outsides that get the finger and lipstick marks; the insides are easy.

—*Judith*

HOW TO DEODORIZE YOUR MICROWAVE

Put in a bowl of water with half a sliced lemon and cook on High for three minutes.

—*Rosa*

HOW TO EASILY CLEAN A DISGUSTING MICROWAVE

Put some washing-up liquid into a jug of cold water and put it in the microwave on High for three or four minutes, depending on just how disgusting it actually is. After the time is up, you will be able to easily wipe all the gunk off just using a cloth and some warm water.

—*Kate*

HOW TO KEEP YOUR KITCHEN SPONGE FROM BREEDING BACTERIA

Put the sponge in your dishwasher every time you run it.

—*frankiegpizza*

HOW TO CLEAN BRUSHED STAINLESS-STEEL APPLIANCES

Clean first with a soft cloth and soapy water, then use baby oil on a cotton pad to polish it when dry.

—*tolgyesikara*

HOW TO CLEAN YOUR DISHWASHER

Just put a handful of washing soda in the bottom of the dishwasher, set it on the hottest cycle, making sure the machine is empty, of course, and go.

—*sandrak*

HOW TO CLEAN A KNIFE BLOCK

Wrap a blunt-ended knife in an antibacterial wipe to clean the slots.

—*leggbarbara*

HOW TO REMOVE BALLPOINT-PEN INK FROM FABRICS

Hairspray really gets rid of ballpoint-pen ink. Just drench the mark with hairspray and you will see it start to lift off. Then rinse with cold water.

—*Mya*

Soak the stain in milk. Just pour some milk into a bowl and put the stained area in, making sure it is covered by the milk. Leave for as long as possible, overnight even, and then wash as normal and your stain will disappear.

—LesleyJ

HOW TO PREVENT POLLEN STAINS FROM FORMING ON FABRICS

Don't go near them with water! Gently blow off any pollen, then roll some Scotch tape, sticky side out, around your fingers and use the tape to gently dab off the pollen. Keep rotating the tape and dabbing until it all comes away.

—NicoleS

The moment your floral arrangement is in the vase, get some tissue and scissors, snip off the ends of the stamens into the tissue, and toss in the bin—you can avoid the nasty stuff altogether.

—eva123

HOW TO GET GREASE MARKS OUT OF SUEDE

Use fuller's earth—it's made of clay so it soaks those stains right up.

—Rosa

HOW TO REMOVE OLD SWEAT STAINS

If the stained shirt is cotton, then soak the area in lots and lots of soluble aspirin in water. Then wash as normal.

—Caroline

HOW TO REMOVE FRESH SWEAT STAINS

Add 1 cup of white vinegar to a bucket (or sinkful) of warm water. Soak your clothes for a couple of hours before laundering as usual. Do not use this method on dry-clean-only clothing.

—*iridescentfaith*

Soak in vodka.

—*Ilana*

HOW TO STOP PILLOWCASES FROM GETTING STAINED WITH FACE CREAM

If you lightly starch your pillowcases, it will help prevent face creams from staining them.

—*Jennifer*

HOW TO REMOVE PERMANENT-MARKER STAINS

Nail-polish remover works for removing marker stains from skin, tables, etc.

—*Brunettebombshell*

HOW TO REMOVE STAINS FROM MARBLE

You can remove stains from marble with a paste of baking soda, water, and lemon juice. Rinse with plain water.

—*Maeve*

HOW TO REMOVE BLOOD FROM FABRICS

If you dip the affected area in milk (any kind!), the blood stain will break down and will come out in a normal washing machine cycle.

—*charleywilde*

HOW TO REMOVE PET-ACCIDENT STAINS

If your pet makes a mess on the floor and you're out of pet-stain remover, simply combine 6 parts water with 2 parts baking soda and 1 part vinegar—rub on the spot and then soak it up.

—*Hillary*

HOW TO REMOVE A RED-WINE STAIN

Most sources suggest either salt, soda water, or white wine. Their effectiveness depends on the pungency of the red wine and whatever it has been spilled on. Always soak up any excess as quickly as possible, then sprinkle with salt before rinsing with cold water or soda water, which should flush away most of the stain. Then wash as usual.

—*nikkiwelch24*

HOW TO REMOVE GRASS STAINS

Blot the stain with distilled malt vinegar before working detergent into the area, then wash as usual. Soaking in glycerine will also remove grass stains from white fabric.

—*nikkiwelch24*

Cream of tartar mixed with water to form a paste removes grass stains when brushed on and left to wash out in the washing machine.

—*soobie*

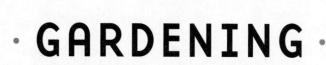

· GARDENING ·

OR SURPRISINGLY PAINFUL BUT STRANGELY REWARDING.

I am a tidying fanatic, so gardening appeals to me enormously. Apart from planting stuff, virtually every task in the garden involves tidying to some degree; mowing the lawn is tidying the grass, pruning is simply tidying a tree, and weeding is the most basic form of tidying there is. Although it's officially classified as a chore, I find weeding tremendously satisfying—you're outside working up a good sweat, and the results are instantly visible. Planting is a different matter, but equally rewarding. As I write, planting a bulb is the closest I've come to giving birth. Realizing that a tulip is living largely because of me fills me with a sense of wonder and pride. And the real joy of most gardening is that it's like paying for a holiday in advance—once the flowers grow, you forget the furiously uncomfortable, backbreaking work of six months earlier.

HOW TO DETER SLUGS

Scatter bark mulch around the base of plants. Apparently prickly surfaces hurt slugs' little paws.

—*Peggy*

Put a bowl of beer at the bottom of the afflicted plant or tree. Slugs and snails love it and will drown in it. Expect to find a full bowl in the morning. Cruel? Maybe, but very effective . . .

—*Mimi*

HOW TO AERATE YOUR LAWN

Forget fancy machines or backbreaking work; just wander up and down wearing your golf spikes.

—*Polly*

HOW TO ATTRACT BIRDS TO YOUR BIRDBATH

If you put the bath near bird feeders, they will naturally use the bath to drink and bathe. Make sure the water is always clean.

—*kimberly1*

HOW TO DISCOURAGE WEEDS AND GRASS
FROM GROWING ON YOUR PATIO

Every so often, pour a bucket of very hot, very very salty water over your patio.

—*Ilana*

HOW TO GET OUT OF TURNING YOUR
COMPOST EVERY FEW WEEKS

Add a handful of worms; they will aerate it for you.

—*Cindy*

HOW TO PERK UP FERNS

You can perk up wilted ferns by watering them once a month with very weak tea.
   —*Valerie*

Use banana peels—just place banana skins around the ferns. There is a lot of goodness in banana skins for plants.
   —*Spatchy*

HOW TO PROTECT YOUR PLANTS, FRUIT, AND VEGETABLES FROM PESTS

Plant marigolds nearby—they seem to deter lots of pests.
   —*Eve*

HOW TO REUSE THE ASH FROM YOUR FIREPLACE

It is great for drying out an overwet compost bin, and it also helps the composting process. I also use the ashes from bonfires.
   —*kimberly1*

HOW TO MAKE COMPOST OF LEAVES AND GRASS CUTTINGS

You can make useful compost in just one season out of a mixture of fallen leaves and grass cuttings, but not of either alone.
   —*Joan*

HOW TO SORT GOOD SEEDS FROM BAD ONES

Pour the seeds into a shallow bucket of water. By morning, the good seeds will have sunk and the bad ones will be floating on top. Be sure to plant the good ones immediately.
   —*Crystal*

HOW TO SOW TINY SEEDS

Use an empty spice shaker to disperse them into the soil.

—*Candace*

HOW TO STOP GARDEN TOOLS FROM RUSTING

Keep them in a bucket of sand.

—*Magda*

HOW TO STOP MOSQUITOES FROM BREEDING IN YOUR WATER BARREL

Pour in a tiny bit of cooking oil.

—*Iola*

HOW TO KEEP YOUR FINGERNAILS CLEAN WHILE GARDENING

Before you start, dig your nails into a bar of soap—it really works.

—*Fawn*

HOW TO DESIGN RAISED VEGETABLE BEDS

Set them at a comfortable working height (not knee height) and make them no wider than allows you to reach to the middle from either side.

—*Zsazsa*

HOW TO GET RID OF DANDELIONS FROM YOUR LAWN

Place a pinch of salt in the center of the rosette of leaves. The plant will die, but be careful not to get salt on the grass or any other plants as it will kill them, too.

—*LadyB*

HOW TO KILL GREENFLY ORGANICALLY

Soak rhubarb leaves in a bucket of water for a few weeks and use the resulting liquid on your plants. Warning: It does really smell!

—*Gwiddon*

HOW TO WEED AMONG DELICATE PLANTS

The best weeding tool is a curved grapefruit knife. With its serrated edge, pointed end, and curved blade, you can extract weeds without hurting delicate plants.

—*Cali*

HOW TO TAKE CARE OF YOUR EYES WHEN GARDENING

When pruning, always cut the branches nearest you first. If you reach past them, your eyes will focus on the back branches and you risk being jabbed, possibly seriously.

—*Cali*

HOW TO WATER YOUR GARDEN POTS MORE EASILY

Take an empty plastic bottle, make small holes all over, and cut off the top to make a wider neck. Place the bottle in the middle of a larger flower pot and surround it with earth, with the neck still exposed. You can now fill up the bottle with water, and the small perforated holes will allow the water to seep into the earth and keep it wet without making a mess. Just keep refilling the bottle with water when the earth is drying out.

—*WATERSIDE*

HOW TO KEEP CATS OUT OF YOUR GARDEN

Sprinkle ground cayenne pepper on the soil every two to three months. This also repels digging dogs, burrowing rodents, and all ants.

—*maryzeee*

HOW TO DETER CATS FROM RELIEVING THEMSELVES IN YOUR GARDEN

I find that mothballs sprinkled around the garden deter felines from using the garden as a litter box.

—*Redlady*

Squirt the little intruders with a water pistol. Cats hate getting wet and won't come back if you douse them a couple of times. It may sound cruel, but it has worked in my garden.

—*Anita123*

HOW TO MAKE FLOWERING BRANCHES LAST IN THE VASE

Cut them at an angle, and then hammer the heck out of the bottom 4 to 6 inches (I do this outside, in our driveway, using a rock and pounding the bottom portion of the branch directly against the asphalt—no clean-up necessary). This splays out the wood so that the branch can suck up water more efficiently. If you don't do this, they won't even look good in the vase for a full day. If you try this, you'll see that they look good for three to five days in the vase.

—*CeeVee*

HOW TO MAKE FLOWERS STAND UPRIGHT IN A VASE

Criss-cross the top of your vase with clear tape, creating lots of squares. Place the stems in all the holes; the tape stops them from falling over. You can put two or three in each hole depending on the size of the opening. This helps the flower arrangement to look very professional.

    —WATERSIDE

Try putting some plastic wrap around the top of the vase and poke the flowers through.

    —COLIYTYHE

To keep roses and tulips upright, pierce a pin through the stem approximately 1 inch down from the flower. When the flower is cut, it can cause an "air lock" in the stem, and when the "air lock" reaches the bloom, it stops food from getting to the flower head.

    —Elaine

HOW TO KEEP CUT FLOWERS FRESH

Put a dash of bleach into the water in a flower vase. It keeps the water clear and slime free, and means you never have to refresh it.

    —Carmen

HOW TO KEEP HOUSEPLANTS SHINY

Polish their leaves by rubbing them with milk mixed with a little water.

    —Judi

HOW TO KEEP CUT ROSES FRESH

Trim the stems of the roses, then plunge the stems into boiling water, counting up to thirty or until you can't see any more air bubbles coming from the stems. I've kept roses for up to three weeks using this method.

—aswas

· COOKING ·

OR SERVING FOOD AT A DIFFERENT TEMPERATURE THAN IT WAS WHEN YOU BOUGHT IT DOESN'T COUNT.

COOKING at its most rewarding is low investment-high yield. These tips will help you be your best self when cooking. And if you cook cleverly, you can entertain simultaneously, instead of being an exhausted, sweaty wreck. While cooking satisfies many women's maternal instinct to feed, the ceremony of food can be quite wearing for the cook and the cookees. Half the secret of cooking is to appear to glide above the surface like a swan—never let them see your feet frantically paddling beneath the water. If people sense you're hysterical, they'll taste it. And if everything doesn't turn out quite as planned, take the advice of one tipster and encourage your guests/family/victims to eat with their mouths, not their eyes.

HOW TO GET AN ONION OR GARLIC
SMELL OFF YOUR HANDS

Rub your hands against anything stainless steel—i.e., a spoon—with dishwashing soap under cool/lukewarm water. Fancy kitchen stores sell stainless-steel "bars" that look like traditional soap for this purpose; however, there is really no need to invest in that when a regular old spoon does the trick.

—*DezG*

If you have a metal sink, run your hands along the rim or the faucet with the water running.

—*missemer*

HOW TO NOT SHRED YOUR FINGERS
ON A CHEESE GRATER

Wear a rubber kitchen glove. It will be grated before your fingers!

—*patsharp*

HOW TO BAKE SUCCESSFULLY

Before you start, have all your ingredients ready and at room temperature. It will make your life a lot easier.

—*Lauren*

HOW TO BEAT EGGS

Adding a little water to the eggs you are beating makes them lighter and less hard work.

—*Regina*

HOW TO FAKE HOMEMADE MAYONNAISE

To impress your guests with homemade-tasting mayonnaise, add fresh lemon (or lime) juice and capers or thyme to ordinary mayo. This makes a tasty spread for sandwiches, grilled fish, or poached chicken.

—*Deborah*

HOW TO GET ALL THE HONEY AND OTHER STICKY STUFF OUT OF A MEASURING CUP

Normally sticky stuff ends up coating the measuring cup, so you end up with less than you thought in the recipe. So very, very lightly oil the measuring cup before you pour in the honey.

—*Zenobia*

Dip the measuring cup in boiling water before you pour in the sticky stuff. It will then slide off easily.

—*joesaunt*

HOW TO REMOVE FAT FROM A STEW

If you have time, leave the stew to cool completely; the fat will be at the top of the dish and you can scoop it off. If you haven't got time, then put stale, hard bread on the top—it will soak up most of the fat.

—*HeatherGrace*

HOW TO UNBROWN ONIONS OR GARLIC

When browning onions or garlic, if they get a bit more toasted than you'd like, simply add a tablespoon of water to your skillet; the brown edges will disappear.

—*Alessandra*

HOW TO GET MORE JUICE OUT OF A LEMON

If you gently heat lemons before squeezing them, you get a lot more juice.

—*Kimberley*

HOW TO TEST IF AN EGG HAS GONE BAD

Fill a pan with water. Bad eggs will float to the top; good ones lie flat on the bottom.

—*Chelsea*

Hold the egg to your ear and shake it. If the egg is fresh, you should not be able to hear the contents slurping around.

—*scifidiva*

HOW TO STOP EGGS FROM CRACKING WHEN BOILED

Pierce a tiny hole in one end of the egg with a very sharp knife before you put it in the water. That will allow any air to escape as it expands, rather than cracking your egg.

—*Kaitlyn*

HOW TO MAKE THE PERFECT POACHED EGG

Before cracking your eggs into a pan of simmering water, gently place each uncracked egg into the water for about twenty seconds. Take these out of the water, stir the water to create a whirlpool, then crack the eggs into it. Placing the eggs uncracked in the water first binds the egg white together so that you have a nice rounded poached egg instead of egg white spreading throughout the whole pan.

—*jojo28*

HOW TO STOP MILK FROM BURNING

Put a large marble in the pan. The marble automatically stirs the milk and prevents it from burning.

—Tracy

HOW TO BUY FISH

Make sure the eyes are still clear. Cloudy eyes mean the fish has been out of the water a few days.

—pippinpuss

HOW TO KEEP LETTUCE FRESH

Add a paper towel to the bag. It will absorb the moisture and keep the lettuce from going slimy too soon.

—Frida

HOW TO DRY LETTUCE

If you want to dry the lettuce after washing it and before using it, put it on the middle of a tea towel, join all four corners together and hold on to them, go outside, and spin the tea towel around over your head or with your arm doing big circles. This removes lots of excess water from the lettuce and the kids love watching you in case you let go of one of the corners.

—COLIYTYHE

HOW TO TOSS A REALLY LARGE SALAD

Throw all the ingredients into a large trash bag. Hold the top and shake.

—kathyleventhal

HOW TO KEEP THE FRIDGE SMELLING SWEET

Wash the inside with a mild bleach solution every couple of months.

—*Myrtle*

HOW TO STOP A CHOPPING BOARD FROM SLIDING AROUND

Putting a wet piece of kitchen towel under a cutting board stops it from sliding around your kitchen countertop.

—*pgrier*

HOW TO STOP AVOCADO FROM GOING BROWN IN A SALAD

Put the pit into the salad bowl until you're ready to serve. This will keep the avocado green. (It also works for guacamole.)

—*LittleBear*

HOW TO STOP A PAN FROM BOILING OVER WHEN MAKING PASTA OR RICE

Place a wooden spoon across the pan and the bubbles will not rise above it.

—*LevantineLass*

Add a splash of olive oil to the water. The oil floats on top and weighs down the bubbles. You can do this beforehand or as it's about to bubble over.

—*Nadienne*

HOW TO REMOVE A BURNED-ON BLACK
STAIN FROM A SAUCEPAN

Soak it overnight with a dishwasher tablet to remove the black burn stain.

—*LadyHelenTaylor*

Fill it with cola and leave it overnight—wash in the morning and the stain will all come off.

—*janhumphries*

HOW TO KEEP PLASTIC WRAP FROM SNARLING

Keep it in the freezer. This seems to give the wrap just enough body and structure to allow it to be rolled off, sheared, and placed over anything without curling up.

—*Abellamiento*

HOW TO MAKE ANY COOKIE CHEWY

I typically bake cookies using butter, but I've learned that if you substitute a little bit of shortening in place of part of the butter, it makes the cookies softer and chewier. If the recipe calls for, say, 2 sticks of butter, you could try $1\frac{1}{2}$ sticks of butter and $\frac{1}{4}$ cup of vegetable shortening.

—*ListenGirlies*

Instead of using softened butter, *melt* the butter over very low heat. This will give you chewy, rather than cakey, cookies.

—*CeeVee*

HOW TO MAKE PERFECT WHIPPED CREAM

Place a bag of frozen peas or corn beneath the bowl. The cold makes the cream whip faster.

—*fashionvictim*

HOW TO MAKE PERFECT PIECRUST

Use frozen, grated butter or shortening instead of butter or shortening that's only been chilled.

—*CeeVee*

HOW TO EXTEND THE LIFE OF A BANANA

Contrary to popular opinion, bananas can be kept in the fridge once they have become yellow and ripe. Although the skin will become black, the fruit itself will remain the same for up to a week. I have done this for years.

—*AudreyT800*

HOW TO PREPARE A CAKE PAN

Whether or not the recipe tells you to, grease *and* flour the cake pan. It makes removing the cake a zillion times easier.

For a chocolate cake, don't use flour ... instead, "flour" the greased pan with unsweetened cocoa. It works perfectly, and you won't have weird white streaks on the cake when you remove it from the pan!

—*CeeVee*

HOW TO NEATLY SLICE CHEESECAKE

Use dental floss (waxed or not). Wrap it around your fingers and gently work it down through the cheesecake. Just make sure the floss is not flavored.

    —CeeVee

HOW TO EXPAND CAKE FROSTING

When you buy a container of cake frosting from the store, whip it in your mixer for a few minutes. You can double it in size. You get to frost more cake/cupcakes with the same amount. You also eat fewer sugar/calories per serving.

    —Lauren32

HOW TO CUT A PIZZA

No pizza cutter? Use a pair of scissors instead.

    —Ursie

HOW TO CUT OPEN A PASSION FRUIT

Don't cut the fruit in half; cut it near the top, as you would a soft-boiled egg. That way you can scoop out the passion fruit pulp with a teaspoon rather than lose most of it on the cutting board.

    —dimlay

HOW TO STOP SALT FROM CLOGGING UP THE SALTSHAKER

Put a few grains of uncooked rice in with the salt. They will absorb moisture but are too big to come out of the holes when using the shaker.

    —Natalie

HOW TO SLICE AN ONION WITHOUT CRYING

This sounds really bizarre, I know—but suck on a teaspoon while chopping. It does work.

—*pearlgirl*

Light a candle near where you are chopping—it burns off the fumes that make you cry.

—*vernbug*

HOW TO ALWAYS HAVE LEMON WEDGES HANDY

To store a ready supply of lemon wedges for drinks, fish, and cooking, slice and deseed lemon slices, roll one by one in a long strip of freezer wrap, and freeze. Individual slices don't stick to each other, defrost in minutes, and are even better in drinks than flabby fresh ones.

—*violet*

HOW TO PREVENT FREEZER BURN

To prevent freezer burn on poultry bones/giblets/scraps you want to save for stock, place each batch in a plastic container, cover with water, and freeze. When ready to use, simply run hot water over the container to loosen, then pop the frozen block into a pot with bay leaf, carrot, celery, onion, and more water, if needed.

—*Cindy*

HOW TO PERK UP STALE BREAD

Place it in a plastic bag and pop it into the microwave for a couple of seconds.

—*mobaskett*

HOW TO RIPEN AVOCADOS

Place them in a fruit bowl with apples. The acid released from the apples helps them ripen easily.

    —pixieflame

Place them in a brown paper bag with a banana.

    —Truthistops

HOW TO GET THE WHOLE STALK OUT OF AN ICEBERG LETTUCE

Holding the lettuce in both hands, tap it firmly and sharply down onto a work surface or a chopping board, stalk side down. The stalk should then be very easy to pull out between your thumb and forefinger.

    —LittleBear

HOW TO STORE CHEESE

Once I have opened a package of grated cheese, I freeze it and use it straight from the freezer for toppings on pizzas, lasagnes, etc. You could grate a block of cheese and freeze the result. This obviously only works for hard cheese.

    —Geedee

If you store cheese in a plastic bag with a sugar cube, it will not mold.

    —Kmzprig

HOW TO CREATE A MEAL PLAN

I've found that posting a weekly menu on my bulletin board in the kitchen is very helpful. It's helpful for older children because they are responsible for feeding themselves breakfast and lunch, and this tells them what food is available for that purpose. It's helpful for teenage boys because they always seem convinced that they are on the brink of starvation and are constantly asking what they will be eating for the next meal (I no longer need to say a word; I just point to the board). It helps me to plan for my errand day, which includes grocery shopping, and it cuts out a lot of waste.

—*Sandrasimmons*

HOW TO STOP CUT POTATOES FROM BROWNING

Keep them in a pan of water till you are ready to use them.

—*Floris*

HOW TO COOK MERINGUES SO THAT THEY ARE CRISP ON THE OUTSIDE BUT SOFT IN THE MIDDLE

Cook them very slowly, in a really low oven. And add a bit of brown sugar, as well as white, to the egg whites—it gives them a lovely golden color.

—*operatix*

Adding a teaspoon of vinegar to the mix will give the baked meringue a lovely squidgy center.

—*Redlady*

HOW TO BUTTER CRACKERS
WITHOUT BREAKING THEM

Simply butter them on top of a piece of bread. Works every time.

—*Pinkdiamond*

HOW TO PEEL AN ORANGE

I score around the top, take off that lid, and score into quarters. No mess. You can also make fun teeth with the quartered peel: With the pith side out, score horizontally, fold slightly back, insert into mouth, and smile.

—*clinic2316*

HOW TO PEEL A MANGO

Don't bother. Hold it lengthways at the narrowest part and slice the sides off as close to the stone as possible. Make vertical and horizontal cuts across the inside of the side pieces, but don't go through the skin. Turn the sides inside out to produce a cubed mango-hedgehog. The cubes can be eaten with the skin still on (messy but fun) or removed one by one with a knife. The fruit on the central oval is best chewed with the rind removed.

—*Lemming*

HOW TO STOP POTATOES FROM SPROUTING

Keep them in a paper (not plastic) bag with an old apple. The chemicals released by the apple as it ages prevent the potatoes from sprouting.

—*Lesley998*

HOW TO KEEP CHIPS FROM GOING STALE

Keep them in the freezer. Most have too much salt to actually freeze, but they won't go soggy from the grease because it's too cold.

—*Persephone*

HOW TO KEEP THE FIZZ IN CHAMPAGNE

Put a metal teaspoon in the bottle. The champagne will still be fizzy the next day!

—*clobee*

HOW TO HAVE A SUCCESSFUL DINNER PARTY

Do not make things you have not made before.

Remember, if it sucks, all things can be purchased and pizza can be ordered, and no one will care. Think of Bridget Jones and the blue soup.

Always leave one or two simple things until the last minute. Someone always shows up early, and giving them a cucumber to chop or a drink to mix puts them at ease and helps you out, too. (I like letting the men light the candles; they like the fire.)

—*onewanderingsoul*

· PETS ·

or The closest thing to being a parent, without the hassle of finding a partner.

As well as the unconditional love thing and all the medically proven health benefits to owning a pet, the main advantage is that they're sensational icebreakers. An awkward social encounter can be eased by admiring your host's charming cats, or by turning the conversation to stories of your dog's naughtiness. Like babies, pets can be wheeled out to be admired, but unlike babies, they can be left alone when you want to go out for dinner. And they'll still love you when you get home. My mother and step-father have two dogs, and such is our family's devotion that while you may see two dachshunds, we see two slightly hairy siblings.

HOW TO GET MORE LOOSE HAIR OUT OF A MOLTING PET

Take a metal wide-toothed comb and a large rubber band; starting at one end, wind the elastic band in and out of the teeth. The elastic grips loose hair much more efficiently, taking you less time to groom your pet, and, also, it does not hurt either of you!

—chrissi70

HOW TO SHAMPOO A DOG

Always wet and shampoo your dog's head last, as this is what makes him shake.

—doingmybest

HOW TO MAKE SURE YOUR DOG IS VISIBLE AT NIGHT

Get a small bicycle reflector and attach it to his collar if he is prone to walking about at night.

—Iris

HOW TO GET RID OF FLEAS

Try eucalyptus oil. Fleas hate eucalyptus.

—Jillaroo95

HOW TO GET SKUNK SMELL OUT OF A DOG

I know it sounds really silly, but I used to work at a veterinary clinic . . . and we always used a douche. This seriously works. There is something about the water, vinegar, and other chemicals that seems to do the trick!

—Mel81

I work at a grooming shop. Our bather uses mouthwash on dogs that have been sprayed by skunks.

—*Estxcami*

HOW TO GET BURRS OUT OF A DOG'S COAT

Put on a pair of rubber gloves for a good grip and work baby oil into the burs; they should slide out more easily.

—*Scout*

HOW TO PROTECT YOUR DOG FROM OTHER DOGS

If your dog regularly gets attacked by other mutts, and especially if you live in an area where many owners don't bother with leashes, carry a fast-unfurling automatic umbrella with the latch undone. If you do get some creature flying at your pooch, you can fend it off (or with luck, frighten it away completely) by opening the umbrella, without any harm being done. There will be nothing for the other owner to object to.

My rescue greyhound had significant fear issues around other breeds, which made him a magnet for aggressive loose dogs, and this protected us many times.

—*Nova7*

HOW TO STOP A PUPPY FROM CRYING EVERY TIME HE IS LEFT ON HIS OWN

The best thing to do is to put a ticking clock and a hot water bottle into a cushion cover near the puppy; the water bottle gives the warmth of your puppy's mother and the ticking replaces the sound of her heartbeat. Worked with mine.

—*Toptip*

HOW TO GET RID OF THE PET SMELL
IN THEIR BEDS AND BLANKETS

Add baking soda to the laundry cycle.

—*Odessa*

HOW TO KEEP YOUR DOG FROM
JUMPING UP AT GUESTS

Tell your guests *not* to do the following:

1. Make eye contact with the dog.

2. Speak to the dog.

3. Allow the dog to "land" on them when he jumps up.

4. Speak or stroke the dog until it is sitting down.

—*WalkinOnSunshine*

HOW TO INTRODUCE A KITTEN TO A NEW HOME

Never let the cat out of the bag! It's a tough task, but put your new kitten in a room you don't use all the time, like a spare bedroom, together with its food, water, and litter tray and leave it there for a day. It will be calm and happy in its new environment and won't run out the door the minute you open it.

—*Eileen*

Put butter on the kitten's paws—it will lick the butter off and pick up the scent of your home as it walks around—that way it will settle in more quickly. Also works for older cats when moving house.

—*Jonahkat*

HOW TO STOP CATS FROM SCRATCHING
THE FURNITURE

If you don't want your cats climbing on your leather sofa or tables, clean them with orange polish—they hate the smell and won't come near it.

    —*Bijou*

Watch your cats closely to see what kinds of things they scratch naturally—furniture, bedding, soft blankets, wood floors, walls. Then purchase an item that has a similar orientation (horizontal/vertical/diagonal) and material as the thing that they like to scratch. This worked like a charm once with a cat that liked to scratch the banisters of stairs. Instead of buying a fancy scratch post, we just bought a bundle of fire wood!

    —*Mally313*

HOW TO SAFELY GIVE PILLS TO CATS

If you have tried wrapping your cat in a towel but find that random claws still escape, try putting your cat inside the sleeve of a sweater (but not one that is very small or tight). Once the cat's head is exposed from the end of the sleeve, pills can be administered. When finished, release the cat by holding the sleeve end open.

    —*Monkeyface*

Crush the tablet or halve it and put it in the cat's food. It's best to hand-feed the food with the tablet in so that you are sure that the cat's had the medicine; plus this avoids stress (and injury) for you.

    —*Babilicious220*

HOW TO TRAIN POSITIVELY UNRULY CATS WHO OPEN CUPBOARDS AND DRAWERS

Double-stick tape is the answer—they hate the tackiness and will avoid it. Works on furniture where they scratch as well. Trust me on this one.

—*Knd*

Try putting aluminum foil on the handles. They hate the noise and the feel. Don't yell at them; it will only make them mad and they won't understand it.

—*Kathyjo*

HOW TO GET RID OF CAT SMELLS IN THE HOUSE

I use a UV light that can be bought at most hardware stores. Switch off all lights; and when you use the UV light, you can find exactly where the cat has been. I have found that window cleaner spray is the best as it breaks down the smell. Saturate the area and rub it with a towel.

—*Macn33*

Make up a solution of warm water, lemon juice, and bicarbonate of soda and spray around the areas that smell of the cat. It neutralizes odors and isn't overpowering like air freshener.

—*Faystevenson*

HOW TO FIND A LOST CAT

Advertise in the local press, circulate fliers around the neighborhood, put notices on lampposts, check with local vets (the cat may have had an accident and been taken there by an animal lover). Animal charities keep lost-and-found registers. Keep faith; cats often go missing and then turn up right as rain.

—*Hmtgeorge*

HOW TO REMOVE TICKS

Forget cigarette ends, etc. Ticks attach themselves by screwing themselves in clockwise. To remove them, just grasp the body and unscrew, counterclockwise.

—*Animalclare*

HOW TO GET OVER THE DEATH OF A BELOVED PET

It took me a long, long time to get over the death of my old pony; I'd had her for nearly thirty years. Take your time and don't feel guilty about still crying over him; you loved him and it's natural. Could you bear to do some volunteer work in an animal rescue center in honor of his memory or do some fund-raising for a local animal rescue center? Maybe you could arrange to plant a tree in a special place, which you can look after and nurture. When I lost my young son, fund-raising for the hospitals that cared for him really helped me—I found it a great therapy and comfort to use life experiences to help others.

—*COLIYTYHE*

HOW TO GET A BIRD BACK INTO ITS CAGE

We had a mynah bird for twenty years, and bribing him with food worked most of the time. But sometimes the only way to get him back was to throw a towel or cloth over him. This always made him stay still for a few moments, enough to gather him up and pop him (plus cloth) back into the cage. We'd remove the cloth when he had settled.

—*josie*

HOW TO NOT LOSE YOUR HORSE IF YOU FALL OFF

Put dog tags on the saddle and bridle with two contact numbers (one on each side).

—*Gwiddon*

HOW TO GET HORSES' STIRRUPS GLEAMING

Put them in the dishwasher.

—*Gwiddon*

HOW TO GET RID OF GREEN ALGAE IN RABBITS' WATER BOTTLES

Put a few grains of uncooked rice with some clean water in the bottle. Replace the lid and shake well. Empty the water and rice and your bottles will look like new. Just check that no rice grains have gone into the tube on the lid as they will restrict water flow.

—*wonderwoman*

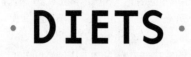

· DIETS ·

or Anything you eat standing up doesn't count, anything liquid doesn't count, and broken cookies don't count because all the calories leak out.

DIETS should not be talked about. They bring out the worst in women. So if you're interested in diets, are on a diet, or have just blown your diet, read this and shut up. Whenever I bang on about being fat, my brother points out that if I really cared that much, I'd do something about it. Harsh but fair. Of course, merely making the decision to go on a diet is guaranteed to make you experience an almost psychedelic hunger, the likes of which you never thought possible. Which inevitably makes you believe it's a fascinating topic of conversation. It isn't. If you talk about it, you draw people's attention to your ass. Don't advertise your diet; you'll look fat, self-obsessed, and neurotic. The most effective dieters are the ones who just get on with it.

HOW TO STICK TO A DIET

Stop beating yourself up. You will "cheat." Most people start a diet, cheat, and then say, "That's it! The diet's over for good." Instead, acknowledge that you've made an error and make a U-turn. Have you ever been in a car with a GPS system? If you miss a turn, does the computer say, "You [fat] idiot! I can't believe you missed that turn [ate fifty-seven cookies!]"? No, the computer says, "Please make a U-turn." It offers no judgments, just gentle instruction. Dieters must do this as well.

—*sandrasimmons*

Like a recovering alcoholic, take it one day at a time. Say to yourself, "For today, I won't eat any chocolate." It's far less scary than thinking you'll never eat chocolate again, and as the days pass, doing without it will become a habit. And there's nothing more habit forming than a habit.

—*Natalie*

HOW TO LOSE WEIGHT BY EATING

A friend of mine told me her aunt lost sixty pounds in a year by simply eating what she wanted but only eating half her regular portion.

—*Palacinka*

HOW TO EAT LESS

To see if you're really still hungry or just being greedy, say to yourself, "If I'm still hungry, I can have more of what I just ate, rather than a dessert." If that isn't so appealing, you know you're being greedy. In fact, a good way to eat less is to just eat a big plate of all one thing. The appetite is stimulated by different flavors, so you'll end up eating less.

—*Jennifer*

It's really simple, but always put your knife and fork down while chewing. It makes you eat *way* more slowly and therefore you feel fuller having eaten less.

—*Marina*

HOW TO PAINLESSLY CURB YOUR APPETITE

Drink water! I keep a small bottle of water at my desk and drink it all day long. The small bottle is key because it doesn't seem like an overwhelming amount, plus it gets you off your ass to refill.

—*rgmontgomery*

Prepare hard-boiled eggs in advance and just have them around to snack on. Also, steamed vegetables, when cold, are delicious.

—*LevantineLass*

HOW TO JUMP-START YOUR WEIGHT LOSS

Keep a diary of every single thing you put in your mouth, including drinks. It can be kind of scary how quickly it adds up.

—*Indira*

HOW TO STOP YOURSELF FROM SNACKING

When there's nothing on television, all you feel like doing is eating, right? Well, what I do is give myself a manicure—as you can't eat with wet nails! You'll stay slim and get gorgeous nails.

—*blondiesuz*

Brush your teeth or rinse your mouth with mouthwash—nothing tastes good after you have done that.

—*amstay*

Knit! You can't eat while knitting—and messy fingers make for messy yarn, so you can't even nibble and knit alternately. Even if all you're capable of is a good old plain stitch, you can liberate all your friends' leftover wool and knit small squares that you can then stitch up into a lovely sofa blanket for cold nights or chilly mornings.

—PoshPaws

A little snacking on veggies, whole fruit (not juice), and whole grains doesn't hurt. The suggestion to have stuff ready to go in the fridge is excellent, but the big thing is to make sure you don't have *any* naughty snacks in your home or at the office. If it isn't there, you can't eat it.

—lmwhthd

Instead of three large meals, eat fist-size meals every three hours. Spread your caloric intake over six meals instead of three. Include a small piece of protein with each meal. You will never feel hungry. I lost twenty pounds by doing this.

—laureah21

HOW TO MAKE YOUR WEEKLY
CHOCOLATE BAR LAST LONGER

Don't you hate it when your weekly chocolate bar (which you allow yourself during your diet) is scoffed down so fast that you can't even taste it? An easy solution to this is to freeze it first; then when you go to eat it, you have to really suck on it and thaw it to taste it.

—seksykt

Make a list of things that you like about yourself, and not just the physical things. Are you just your body or do you value your other assets? When you think of the things you don't like about your body, are they things that can change with diet and exercise? Think of three people you admire. Is it only their bodies you find attractive? Your body is always a work in progress; worry about keeping your heart open and your mind alert.

—*Masi*

HEALTH AND FITNESS

OR PIZZA IS NOT AN APPROPRIATE BREAKFAST FOOD.

LOOKING at fitness from my not-particularly-fit perspective, it appears to be a necessary evil. At some point in your life a situation will arise when you have to hurry for something, swim to a boat, or walk up a hill in the company of other sentient beings. If you are able-bodied and allow yourself to get so unfit that these things are beyond you, it's a sign of idiocy, like racism or bigotry. If you wish to be taken seriously, you simply have to be mobile. The sheer humiliation of being puffingly unfit in these mundane circumstances is enough to drive most of us to the gym every once in a while. That, and finally understanding that if you're over thirty and want to continue eating anything that even faintly resembles happiness, you're going to have to pay a price somewhere.

HOW TO IMPROVE YOUR BALANCE AND POSTURE

Think of your nipples as headlights and keep them lighting the way ahead, not the road at your feet!

    —*Yvonne*

I have friends who are models, and the way they are taught to walk is: ears behind shoulders and shoulders behind hips. It takes a bit of practice, but it will be second nature in no time.

    —*murph*

Adjust your computer chair so it sits as low as is still comfortable. This way, you are never tempted to slouch and you look straight ahead at the computer screen.

    —*Brenna*

HOW TO GET RID OF A STY IN YOUR EYELID

This may seem really strange, but I remember when I was very young, the older folks used to say to rub a gold ring over the sty. I don't know whether it was coincidence or not, but it worked.

    —*nala*

HOW TO KNOW HOW LONG YOU SHOULD BRUSH YOUR TEETH

If you want to know how long you should brush your teeth, imagine singing "Happy Birthday" to yourself twice over. It cheers the morning up no end. And you should get into the habit of doing Kegel exercises at the same time.

    —*Kerry*

HOW TO NOT CATCH A COLD

Wash your hands—*a lot*—and stop touching your face. You pick up masses of germs by touching things and then touching your eyes, nose, and mouth—these are all great entry points for germs.

—*Golda*

HOW TO EAT MORE FRUIT

I freeze fresh fruit—blueberries and raspberries (in resealable freezer bags)—then add the frozen berries to my cereal; it keeps the milk cold.

—*Bethany*

HOW TO GET TO SLEEP *AND* BE A HAPPIER PERSON

When you are horizontal, you are not allowed to think about anything that requires a solution. This is the Horizontal Rule—as in the middle of the night your left-side, problem-solving brain is fast asleep and your right-side, drama-queen brain is wide awake. Instead, the only thing you are allowed to do is to count your blessings or think of five things you are grateful for that day. If you are still awake, then think of five things you were grateful for yesterday, and the day before and the day before that and so on. Not only does this actually get you to sleep, it also makes you a happier, nicer person.

—*Gam*

HOW TO GET BACK TO SLEEP

If you suffer from insomnia due to a racing brain, try counting your breaths. If you get distracted and find yourself thinking about something else, start again. You'll soon bore yourself to sleep.

—*Deborah*

I think of a color, and then think of all the things in the world that are that color, and list them in my head. It's ... sooo ... boring ...

—*bangzoom*

Throw off the covers and get really, really cold for about ten minutes or as long as you can stand, then turn onto your side and pull up the covers! Works every time.

—*joesaunt*

HOW TO MANAGE A TOOTHACHE

Instead of loading up on pills, try holding an ice cube on the bit of skin where the base of your thumb meets your forefinger on the same side as your toothache is on.

—*Carissa*

If you cannot get hold of any ice easily, just try pinching the piece of skin between the thumb and forefinger on the same side that your toothache is coming from. This really does work!

—*rosepink*

HOW TO REMOVE A SPLINTER

A splinter comes out much more easily if you soak the whole area in olive oil first.

—*Mallory*

HOW TO STOP A BEE STING FROM STINGING

Once you have removed the stinger, rub the area with a banana peel.

—*Scout*

Don't know how this one works, but if you remove the stinger and then tape a penny over the stung area, it will stop hurting and the swelling and redness will go down in fifteen minutes.

—*Quintella*

HOW TO SOOTHE A JELLYFISH STING

I find that rubbing the area with vinegar—any kind of vinegar—takes away the sting.

—*curvylady*

HOW TO STOP MUSCLE CRAMPS

When you get a cramp in your calf, stretch your leg out and pull your foot up so it's at a sort of right angle with your leg. It goes straight away!

—*leighanneb18*

If you get a cramp in your foot, the best thing to do is stand flat on it and lean against the wall so that you are really stretching out your calf muscle.

—*Leah*

HOW TO TREAT SUNBURN

Add some vinegar to cool water, dip a dish towel in it, and lay it on the sunburn.

—*Redlady*

Apply a few drops of lavender oil to a cotton ball and spread the oil over the skin—the burning sensation will lessen within half an hour.

—*Help123*

Take an antiinflammatory and then soak in a warm bath with a cup of baking soda in it.

    —Shirley

HOW TO KEEP COOL IN A HOT CLIMATE

I live in Florida, *and* I'm postmenopausal and have horrible hot flashes, so keeping cool is a priority with me. A quick cool-off that always works is to wet your hands with cool water and gently rub the water on your arms and legs, the back of your neck, and your face. The rubbing will bring your blood to the surface, where the water will cool it (stand in front of a fan if possible). Also, wear cotton! Polyester and blends don't absorb moisture and make you really hot.

    —asildem

Put a damp cloth under your sun hat.

    —Verity

HOW TO REMEMBER TO DO KEGEL EXERCISES

I do them every time I stop for a traffic light until it turns green. It becomes a habit very quickly once you see the results!

    —coleen

I do mine in the supermarket line. Also when filling my car with gas.

    —Redlady

Do them after you've been to the bathroom. As most people go several times a day, you'll have the muscles strengthened up in no time!

    —ella

If you have a slow Internet connection or often wait for things to download, use this time to do Kegel exercises. You'd only be staring into space anyway.

—*Leah*

※

HOW TO DE-STRESS

Try boxing. Beat the snot out of your least favorite pillow. If violence doesn't appeal to you, try any really heart-pumping cardio. Running and rowing both do it for me. Not only are you working too hard to stay stressed out, but the endorphins these activities create will make you feel better.

—*keryn*

When you're really stressed in a situation, breathe in love and breathe out fear . . . It works!!

—*ElleMacpherson*

Stand up straight, put your hands at your sides, lift them slowly up over your head, and stretch as if you are trying to push the ceiling back in place. Then take a deep breath and exhale with a sigh three times.

—*Masi*

※

HOW TO STOP SMOKING

I used the three-minute rule: When you feel a craving, say to yourself, I'll wait three minutes and then see how I feel. The craving always subsided after the three minutes were up, and I had usually been distracted by something else during the wait. It has been six years since my last cigarette!

—*DawnRaid*

HOW TO STAVE OFF DEPRESSION

Notice the signs, and when your mood starts to drop, see it as a warning sign and start to practice "extreme self care." *Before* you fall all the way to the bottom of the mood pile, do something nice for yourself. Pretend you're a visitor to your neighborhood. Take yourself out for coffee and cake. Pay someone else to make your lunch. Read a paper. Window-shop. Try out perfumes and lip glosses with no intention to purchase. It feels naughty but nice.

—*pinglepops*

HOW TO MAKE YOURSELF DRINK MORE WATER

Put some water in bottles in the fridge; if you measure out your "daily requirement," you can sip or swig as the day goes by and monitor how much you are drinking. Keep the bottles small so that you do not become overwhelmed by the prospect of getting through large bottles. Put in a bit of juice for flavor if necessary.

—*COLIYTYHE*

HOW TO REMEMBER TO TAKE PILLS

I set "Pills" as a daily event in the calendar on my cell phone. That way the alarm goes off at the same time every day and I never forget to take them!

—*bunny*

HOW TO EXERCISE FOR FREE

Meet up with some moms and go for a walk together after dropping the children off at school. With all the chat going on, you hardly notice the exercise. Take a bottle of water with you. If you're walking on your own, stay in populated areas and walk in daylight; try not to put yourself at risk. You could also find out if you have a bike route nearby. You can cycle for miles, safely and for free.

—*COLIYTYHE*

If you travel to work by bus or subway, get off one stop before you usually do and walk the rest of the way. This can eventually be increased to two stops.

Walk up and down stairs instead of using the elevator. You can start by going up stairs for a week, and then down, and then combine both.

—*Finlandia*

HOW TO KEEP TO AN EXERCISE PLAN

Schedule exercise appointments in your planner, so you actively block out the time for them. If you try to just fit them in where you can, *everything* else will take priority.

—*Winifred*

HOW TO START RUNNING (FOR WEIGHT LOSS) IF YOU HATE RUNNING . . .

I find I am much better on a treadmill because it forces you to keep the pace and also is less harsh on your joints. Make sure you put energy-boosting and dance-party tunes on your iPod, and when you're running, imagine you're dancing at a club.

—*AllieN*

HOW TO LOOK LIKE YOU HAVE A FLAT STOMACH AND GET ONE AT THE SAME TIME . . .

Sounds obvious but hold in your tummy as much as you can all the time (even when no one's looking!). I find after a while it really works!

—*josie24*

HOW TO TONE YOUR STOMACH

Sit up straight, pull your stomach in as far as it can go, hold, and count backward from 100. It's harder than you think, but if you work up to doing this eight times a day you'll see the difference.

—*Masi*

Sit upright at your computer; don't rest your back against the chair. Now between your Internet searches or whatever, take a deep breath and hold it for a count of, say, forty or fifty and then exhale. While you're holding the breath, your stomach should feel firm to the touch. Repeat this for many reps and whenever you're just waiting for something and have a few minutes to kill.

—*firefly1*

HOW TO TONE YOUR BUTT

Squeeze your buttocks while watching TV, in quick reps of fifty.

—*Redlady*

HOW TO LOOK GOOD WITH A HANGOVER

The key is (weirdly) to wear less makeup, rather than trying to disguise the effects with more. Your skin will be dehydrated, so moisturize vigorously. Cover up under-eye bags with a light touch, put a bit of healthy-looking pink blusher on the apples of your cheeks, stick to sheer and pale eye shadows, and apply mascara—if your hand isn't shaking too much.

   —*Sharon*

Wear a crisp, white shirt with a collar. It will reflect light onto your face and no one will be the wiser! I used to always keep an ironed white shirt in the closet for such emergencies . . . nothing shows off your hangover quite like a crumpled black shirt.

   —*jennpod*

I have a friend who applies a light self-tanning moisturizer last thing before bed at the end of a big night and wakes up looking sun-kissed and healthy.

   —*Blingrid*

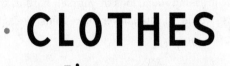

· CLOTHES ·

OR I'M A CHIC AND FABULOUS WOMAN, AND THEN I WAKE UP.

WHETHER you're a Goth or Jackie O, nothing beats clean, pressed clothes worn with confidence. Confidence is key when it comes to dressing successfully. I have a friend who has a far-from-perfect body, yet she wears clothes usually worn by women with phenomenal figures. Her legs could be better, but she wears shortish skirts, and people believe the "code" for "good legs" that they are seeing. In a triumph of presentation over reality, she has ended up with the image of being a babe with a great figure. I'm not suggesting for a moment that you encase your tubbiest bits in Lycra and then expect others to think of you as Cindy Crawford, but the lesson has to be learned: When you wear your "fat clothes," everyone else sees "fat clothes," too.

The best advice my grandmother gave me was: "Just because they make it in your size doesn't mean you should wear it." When you're in the dressing room, look at yourself hard in the mirror and say those words . . . you'll never make a mistake again!

    —vancouvergirl

Buy only clothes that make you want to do a happy dance in the dressing room.

    —benjizoot

I ask myself the question, Do I look better/nicer in the item than in what I was wearing when I went into the dressing room? If the answer is yes, then I'll likely buy it. If it's a relief to take it off and get back into my old clothes, then it's a no!

    —jeyacalder

I try to have the "buy one, throw one" rule. This means that if I buy something, I have to throw something away. If there is nothing in my closet that I would be willing to do without in order to replace it with what I want, then I obviously don't want it that much!

    —princessbella

HOW TO STOP A RUN IN YOUR HOSE

Liquid glue is a good solution if you don't have any clear nail polish. Dab a little glue on the inside edges of the run . . . let the glue dry and that run will not go anywhere.

    —Xandri

HOW TO FIX A HEM

ᢗᢙᢋᢋᠥ

If the hem of your skirt or trousers comes undone, pretty much every office and restaurant in the world has a stapler you can borrow in an emergency. If you're wearing hose, make sure the sharp bits face away from your hose.

—*Trula*

ᢙᢉᢋᢋᠥ

HOW TO REALLY CLEAR OUT YOUR CLOSET

ᢗᢙᢋᢋᠥ

Have a clothes-swap party with your friends; that way you know your unwanted stuff is going to a good home and you end up with some new (to you!) stuff. Think of this as recycling and socializing at the same time.

—*kezzajane*

First, take every single thing out and put it all in piles of similar stuff—only then decide what to chuck. It's easier to be ruthless if you can see that you already own twelve pairs of black trousers.

—*Hillary*

Get someone else to help. My sister and daughter are great; they have no emotional ties to my clothes and have no hesitation telling me if something's past its "sell-by" date or looks awful. I then have space in my small closet, and the thrift shop benefits.

—*Lynda*

1. Empty your entire closet.

2. Try on everything and look at yourself in the mirror.

3. When you return your clothing to the closet, turn all the hangers backward on the rod. Mark a date in your calendar either six months or one year ahead, and when that date comes, take a hard look at those items that are still backward on the rod and realize you will probably never wear

them. Someone else will, though, so pass them on and bless someone else with them.

—*sandrasimmons*

I cleared out my closet when I was really angry—which made me ruthless.

—*ahlh*

HOW TO KNOW WHEN YOU HAVE TOO MANY CLOTHES

Invest in a certain number of "nice" hangers. When you start having to use those wire ones from the dry cleaner, you know it's time for a closet clear out.

—*Gam*

HOW TO ACHIEVE THE PERFECT CLOSET

Organize your closet to reflect your lifestyle—like a pie chart. If the majority of your life is spent at work, then the majority of your clothes should be work clothes (unless you are lucky enough to wear a uniform!). Your weekend and evening clothes should then take the minority of the space and your spangles should take up the least. If you have more going-out clothes than work clothes and you only go out once a year, you're going to look great at work!

—*carriehelen*

HOW TO UNSTICK A ZIPPER

Rub plain white bar soap, like Ivory, on the zipper; it will wax it making it run smoothly.

—*femme*

Rub a lead pencil on either side and it should run smoothly again.

—*MillieFox*

Rubbing a candle along the zipper works as well; the waxiness helps it unstick.

—*ariel1004*

HOW TO FIX A LOOSE THREAD ON A SWEATER

To put a loose thread (or a pulled line) on a fine knitted item back into its place, get a needle and push it through to the other side (i.e., the inside); paint the thread lightly with clear nail varnish. This stops it from coming back out again and is invisible from the outside.

—*ariel1004*

HOW TO LOOK GOOD

I don't really understand the purpose of flat shoes—my top tip for any girl would have to be: Never be seen out of the house in anything other than heels.

—*DonatellaVersace*

HOW TO ALWAYS LOOK PULLED TOGETHER

Always wear lipstick. My mom always told me that I shouldn't leave the house without lipstick, because I look dead without it. It took me too long to realize that she was right!

—*FrancesHouseman*

Take a few minutes before bed to set out your outfit and accessories for the next day. Rushing is the easiest way to ruin your look.

—*CassandraM*

HOW TO AVOID FOUR BUTT CHEEKS

Wear proper-sized, proper-fitted underwear. There's no point wearing a micro string thong if you have a lovely, sexy, curvy, but macro-sized ass.

—*Slothie*

HOW TO SORT AND PUT AWAY SOCKS WHILE HAVING *FUN*

We started Sock Night when our kids were little. I seemed to always have a pile of socks in the laundry room that I procrastinated about and just didn't want to fold. So I thought up a game called Sock Night. Once a week the whole family would sit in a circle and we'd put the mound of socks in the middle. Someone would say "Go!" and then everyone would pick up some socks and throw them at the person to whom they belonged! Once the sock throwing is over, each person folds up their own socks and puts them away. You cannot do this and not laugh. It's just not possible. It's also a good way to get some good conversations going, whether you do this with children or your sweetie. It makes for some wonderful memories.

—*sandrasimmons*

HOW TO CLEAN SUEDE

Use a clean pencil eraser to remove marks.

—*AnyaHindmarch*

HOW TO WASH DOWN-FILLED GARMENTS

Put a tennis ball into the dryer to keep the down properly distributed.

—*Magnolia*

HOW TO STRAIGHTEN OUT A COLLAR OR EDGE OF CLOTHING WITHOUT GETTING OUT THE IRON

Use hair flat irons. They may damage some fabrics, but they work well on cotton tops.

—*janine*

HOW TO MAKE AN EMERGENCY LINT REMOVER

Wind tape, sticky side out, around your hand a few times, and you have an instant lint/pet hair remover.

—*Gam*

· ACCESSORIES ·

OR MEN HAVE TEAM SPORTS,
WE HAVE HANDBAGS.

I am convinced that just as the moon is a magnet for water, diamonds are a magnet for estrogen. Why else would otherwise rational women be rendered a bit giggly in the presence of diamond jewelry? After all, the casual observer can't tell the difference between a diamond and a piece of cut glass, so why all the fuss? The only logical answer is that diamonds have magical powers, kind of like kryptonite. Almost all real jewelry is imbued with a certain magic anyway. We tend to give and receive it at important moments and so it acquires a talismanic quality, way beyond any prosaic value. I own a gold-and-garnet ring that looks like anything you could pick up in an average jewelry shop. Until you realize that it is Hellenistic, which makes it roughly 2,200 years old. Can you imagine what that one ring has meant to so many different women? Now that's magic.

HOW TO ACCESSORIZE

Get dressed as normal, and if you're worried that you've overaccessorized, turn your back to the mirror. Turn around quickly and take off the first thing you see.

—*Justine*

HOW TO POLISH HANDBAGS

Clear aerosol or paste furniture polish is the best polish for leather handbags.

—*AnyaHindmarch*

HOW TO REMOVE WATERMARKS
FROM LEATHER HANDBAGS

I used baby wipes that contain aloe to clean my bag and it worked like a charm. Using a soft, damp cloth with a couple drops of baby oil will also do the trick.

—*maryzeee*

HOW TO BE ORGANIZED IF YOU
USE SEVERAL HANDBAGS

I use several favorite handbags and it is a hassle to keep putting the bare necessities into each one (lip gloss, tweezers, breath freshener, etc.). I keep these in a clear plastic cosmetic bag that fits into all of my favorite handbags, and when I change bags, I just grab the clear bag and pop it in the handbag that I will be using that day.

—*terryleecox*

HOW TO GET OFF A STUCK RING

Apply dish soap to your finger and the ring should come off quickly.

   —ysmith77

Rub margarine or butter around the finger and the ring, and it will help to slide it off.

   —pjamas10

Start by running your hand under very cold water. If that doesn't work, then wind sewing thread tightly and evenly around your finger between the ring and the fingernail—starting closest to the ring. Pass the end of the thread under the ring and pull gently—this will unwind the string and ease the ring off.

   —Bianca

HOW TO CLEAN DIAMONDS

If you are out of jewelry cleaner, try vodka.

   —Jewel

The best thing to use is dishwashing liquid and a soft, old toothbrush. Remember to clean them in a bowl; there will be no way they can be washed down the sink!

   —mmaccaw

HOW TO CARE FOR PEARLS

Apply your perfume, hair spray, creams, makeup, etc. before putting on your pearls. The harsh chemicals can damage the luster. Don't put perfume on your neck if you are wearing pearls. Store them in a soft silk, satin, or velvet pouch; never store them next to metals as they can scratch the pearls. Pearls do love natural body oils, so wear them regularly. Clean them with a soft, damp cloth after a few wears.

—waxy1o86

❧

HOW TO CHECK IF PEARLS ARE REAL OR NOT

Gently rub/tap the pearl against your teeth. If it feels very smooth, it's fake. Real pearls feel slightly gritty.

—waxy1o86

❧

HOW TO CLEAN VINTAGE COSTUME JEWELRY

Please don't ever put rhinestones (vintage or otherwise) into water or chemical dips. Moisture will damage the foil backing, dulling the stones. This can also cause any type of glued-in stone to loosen from the setting.

It's far safer to put a tiny bit of glass cleaner or sudsy water on a soft cloth and gently wipe the jewelry (if simply dusting it doesn't work). Then dry it very quickly with a hair dryer set on cool.

—glitzqueen

❧

HOW TO STORE JEWELRY

If your jewelry is in a mess and all you can see is a big pile, you'll never wear any of it. Store small pieces such as earrings and rings in ice cube trays. They stack easily, too.

—Judith

❧

HOW TO PACK JEWELRY FOR TRAVEL

Save the tiny resealable plastic bags that come on new clothing (with the extra button or thread) and drop your necklaces or earrings into these before stashing them in your travel bag.

—Sundance

HOW TO STOP METAL JEWELRY FROM
TURNING YOUR SKIN GREEN

Paint it with clear nail polish. This works on rings, bracelets, and earrings. It also works if certain metals irritate your skin. I bought an expensive watch with a chain strap and it caused bumps, so I painted all the parts that touched my skin and now I can wear it with no problem.

—livliv

HOW TO STOP LOSING YOUR JEWELRY

If you take off your jewelry to wash your hands in a public bathroom, put it in your mouth. You'll never leave a precious ring in a service station bathroom again.

—Gam

Thread rings through your watch, fasten the catch, and stick it down your bra. If you forget, the weird lump will surely attract comment.

—psbarth47

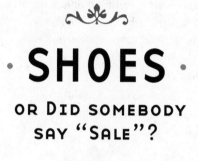

· SHOES ·

OR DID SOMEBODY SAY "SALE"?

CAN anyone tell me a less practical place on the body to put a four-inch nail? The elbow would be inconvenient, but not truly hampering. The kneecap could be dangerous to others, but with due care wouldn't really get in the way of our daily lives. And the shoulder could even be quite chic, in a Flash Gordon sort of a way. Who exactly was the moron who decided that we should attach them to the soles of our feet? What's with this voluntary disability that we think is so irresistibly attractive? Whatever; we've fallen for it, everyone we know has fallen for it, and so we will continue to wear high heels. And not only wear them but be transported to unimaginable ecstasies by a new pair at 50 percent off. Which we will never wear because they hurt. Incredible.

HOW TO BUY SHOES

Always buy shoes after drinking one glass of wine (no more). Then you are a little adventurous but haven't lost your good sense. Come to think of it, you should do nearly everything after just one glass of wine.

—*lolabelle*

Always buy shoes at the end of the day when your feet are at their most swollen.

—*Scarlett*

HOW TO BUY HIGH HEELS

Shift your weight around, try a little jump step, stand on one foot for a few seconds. If you can't do this, then the heels are too high.

After walking around for a few minutes, try walking backward for three steps. If you can do that naturally, without feeling like you're off balance, then you've found a good pair.

—*Masi*

HOW TO WALK IN HIGH HEELS

Two words: *weight back.* (Let your weight rest more on your heels instead of leaning forward and trying to bear your weight on your toes or the balls of your feet.) I have literally stopped people who looked as though they couldn't walk in their heels, told them, and seen them have an "Aha!" moment.

—*Peachy503*

Put one foot directly in front of the other. It makes such a difference and makes you feel sexier when you walk!

—*oojessoo*

HOW TO DEODORIZE SHOES

You can deodorize smelly sneakers and hiking shoes by sprinkling them with baking soda.

    —Chantal

I put fabric softener sheets in the smelly shoes in my household. I don't know how long the various shoes stay fragrant, but it stops my utility room (the home of most shoes) from smelling.

    —Ally1310

HOW TO CLEAN PATENT LEATHER

You can clean patent leather with a cloth dipped in milk. Buff afterward.

    —Bridget

To give your patent leather a lovely shine, put a small smear of Vaseline on a soft cloth and buff.

    —thepoet

HOW TO REPAIR SCUFFED HEELS

If they are a dark color and the plastic heel has been exposed due to scuffs, you can try coloring in the scuff with a black marker pen. I do it to all my shoes, even the Jimmy Choos.

    —Odette

HOW TO SQUEEZE ON TIGHT BOOTS

If you are trying to put on boots and your legs are too clammy or the boots have a rough interior that prevents them from sliding nicely up your leg, put your foot into the point of a plastic shopping bag and pull the boot on over the bag. Once the boot is up smoothly, pull the plastic bag until it breaks, and pull it up and out of the boot.

—*Penelope*

HOW TO STORE BOOTS

Take an old magazine and roll it. Stick the roll inside the leg of the boot—it will keep the top portion of the boot from flopping over in your closet and the ankle portion won't wrinkle or wear away as quickly. Make sure, however, that the magazine you put in one boot is the same size as the one you put in the other. . . .

—*paulinast*

HOW TO AVOID BLISTERS WHILE CAMPING, HIKING, OR BACKPACKING

First put on a cheap pair of knee-high hose and then put on your socks and boots. Instead of your socks rubbing against your skin and creating blisters, the friction ends up between the hose and your socks instead. Voilà: no more blisters.

—*CeeVee*

HOW TO PREVENT BLISTERS

If you're wearing new shoes without tights, coat your feet with Vaseline. You can also use natural lip salve if your shoes start rubbing during the day. No rubbing = no blisters.

—*Gam*

HOW TO STOP SHOES FROM RUBBING

You can rub a dry cake of soap around the offending edge that is rubbing. This will make a nice waxy coating to stop the rubbing and allow you to wear the shoes long enough to soften the leather.

—*Ferny*

HOW TO STRETCH SHOES

To soften leather, cut up a potato and stuff it into the area that you want stretched or softened. Leave the potato overnight. It works; don't ask me how, but it does.

—*Barbaric*

Blow a warm hair dryer on them for twenty or thirty seconds, until they are thoroughly warmed up, then put them on. They should stretch and mold to your feet.

—*triciab1023*

HOW TO CLEAN FLIP-FLOPS

I hate it when the inside soles of my flip-flops get dirty, so I clean them with wet wipes.

—*Luz*

This sounds disgusting, but you can put all-rubber flip-flops in the dishwasher. Just don't dry them on "hot"!

—*Judi*

HOW TO REMOVE THOSE ANNOYING STICKERS FROM THE SOLES OF NEW SHOES

Set your hair dryer to its hottest setting and blast the sticker with hot air for thirty seconds or so. You will find that the glue very quickly starts to soften/melt, allowing the sticker to peel off the sole cleanly and easily, leaving no residue!

This technique can also be used to remove sticky labels from other items when you need to give them as a gift!

—*happyhelper*

· BEAUTY ·

OR THEY SAID THAT ZITS WERE JUST A PHASE. THEY LIED.

WRINKLES and pimples at the same time? Hello? It's enough to make you question the existence of a supreme being. Imagine if the day your first pimple eased its way onto your previously flawless face, you hadn't been gently reassured by someone cooing, "Don't worry, you'll grow out of them." Imagine if instead they'd said, "Yup, you're hosed. These things will continue to blight you—usually on particularly important and romantic occasions—for the rest of your livelong days." But (and this may be proof that the Supreme Being has a sense of humor) there are measures you can take to combat both pimples and wrinkles—although sometimes hearing what other women are doing can lead you to identify problems you didn't even know you had. . . . Hairy arms? I hadn't even noticed my own until a friend told me she'd found a great new brand of bleach. Terrific.

HOW TO WAX YOURSELF

Be committed to it. Don't kid yourself; it will hurt. Pulling slowly or less violently will not make it less painful. It will just pull off skin or cause irritation. Be committed to ripping it off—despite the sound and pain.

—Slothie

Make sure you hold down the skin at the bottom of the wax strip so that the area you are ripping wax off is taut. This will ensure that the strip is pulled off quicker without taking half your leg or bikini area with it! Ouch!

—Hussy

HOW TO PREPARE FOR A BIKINI WAX

Exfoliate like your life depends on it a week before your appointment.

—TraceyMichelle

Take a painkiller an hour before, and it won't hurt as bad.

—pklimas

HOW TO RELATIVELY PAINLESSLY WAX YOUR UPPER LIP

Glide an ice cube over the area to numb before and after waxing to soothe and close the hair follicle.

—loobieloo

HOW TO GET THE BEST RESULT WITH SELF-TANNERS

Slather your hands, elbows, knees, and feet with moisturizer before you apply a self-tanner. Immediately afterward wash your hands thoroughly and wipe your knees (back and front), elbows, and ankles.

—Abigail

HOW TO STOP SELF-TANNERS FROM STAINING YOUR SHEETS

If you've just applied a self-tanner and don't want to stain your sheets, get an old duvet cover and sleep inside it with your duvet on top. I always take a duvet cover when I'm sleeping in hotels with bedding that isn't clean enough for my liking.

—Bianca

HOW TO GET RID OF SELF-TANNER STREAKS

I found (accidentally) that cream hair bleach will remove self-tanner streaks. Since it's so thick, it can be placed exactly where you want it. Just leave it on for a couple of minutes, testing to see if it's worked its magic. Then go over the botched area with self-tanner mixed with moisturizer for a softer, blended tan line.

—mcat35

Nail-polish remover works!

—nominoo

Apply whitening toothpaste to the dark area for a short while . . . wash it off and you'll see it diminishes the color. This is also very effective if you've applied self-tanner with bare hands and now have orange palms. Applying whitening toothpaste liberally to your palms for five minutes or so solves the problem!

—Barrkas

HOW TO APPLY PERFUME

Apply perfume once you have washed and moisturized. However, always try to remember this strict rule: If you can still smell your perfume a couple of minutes after applying, you're wearing too much!

—sophie08

Perfume should never be applied so that it remains in a place (e.g., an elevator) when you are no longer there. Ideally, it should be light enough so that one smells it only when close enough to kiss you.

—Pamela

My friend found out that the guy at work she fancied liked Jean Paul Gaultier perfume on women. So when she was ironing her work shirts, she added a tiny amount of perfume into the iron where the water goes. The shirts had a very subtle whiff of fragrance and the man was entranced. She hadn't doused herself in the stuff, but he couldn't work out why she smelled so heavenly. The iron was probably ruined, but she said the attention was worth it.

—ishouldjojo

HOW TO APPLY PERFUME ON THE GO

Rather than carry around a big bottle of perfume, I always ask the sales assistant for a couple of sample testers of my favorite brand whenever I'm stocking up.

—Kelsey

HOW TO AVOID RAZOR BUMPS

Buy a big bottle of light conditioner for hair. Use it in the shower to shave your legs. It works better than shaving lotion or soap and leaves your legs soft and smooth.

    —maresydotes

I find the most vital part of shaving overall is exfoliating. I used to get terrible shaving rash all over, which I then realized was due to my dry skin—my razor would snag on it. Eventually I got so fed up with it that I bought a sugar rub, which you can get from most beauty shops or supermarkets; I would exfoliate like mad before shaving to make sure my legs were as smooth as could be. Since then my legs have been silky smooth. Exfoliating also prevents ingrown hairs. Exfoliating is possibly the best thing you can do for your skin. It keeps the skin fresh.

    —Irishcharm

HOW TO MAKE YOUR OWN BODY SCRUB

Granulated sugar mixed with your body wash or shampoo makes an amazingly cheap and effective body scrub. I tried it and now have a glass container of sugar in my bathroom. It works better than anything I've ever tried before. I have a really foamy face wash, so I also add sugar to that and it lathers up and scrubs, leaving me super soft and smooth, without oil. I apply my own oil afterward and my bath doesn't get so greasy.

    —Halle

HOW TO PREVENT BACKNE

Put a few drops of tea tree oil in your bath water everyday. The result? *Amazing!* I have suffered back acne all my life; after this my back is flawless.

    —obaseme

When showering, always wash/condition/rinse your hair first and then wash your back. The residue from your hair will stay on your back if you don't wash it off, and this will cause acne.

—*kated*

HOW TO KEEP YOUR BREASTS PERKY AS LONG AS POSSIBLE

I am sixty-three and have really perky breasts. I spray them daily with cold water and do the following exercise: Clasp hands together and push. Do fifty repetitions.

—*Redlady*

HOW TO BEAT CELLULITE

I work in a gym, so I know what's great and what's not worth the time. A machine called a stepper is fantastic and about the best you can get for your bum. If you can manage 10 minutes every 2 days on that, I guarantee miracles in a couple of weeks. A tan can also help, as the dark tone on your skin can cover cellulite.

—*tink*

Don't—get over it. Anyone who judges you by the dimpliness of your thighs isn't worth the bother, and cellulite can't be gotten rid of anyway. You can improve it for a short while, but it is just the body's way of storing fat—in little pockets. Sorry, gals.

—*littlebean*

Don't get mad at your cottage-cheese thighs; pamper them. Get a great-smelling moisturizer with skin-tightening properties; use it daily. And remember that the lighter your skin, the more your least favorite dimples will show, so consider a self-tanner for a little camouflage. Exercise, and drink water. Love yourself, dimples and all!

—*ListenGirlie*

HOW TO STOP CRACKED HEELS

Lather your feet at bedtime with good old Vaseline, with extra coverage on the heels. Put on cotton socks, and the next morning your feet will be like a baby's.

—Lucille

HOW TO GET RID OF YELLOW SKIN ON THE SOLES OF FEET

Get a tomato and cut off the top—the part you usually throw away—then rub it over your calluses. The citric acid will soften them. You need to do this a few times to see results, but it's less dangerous than using a blade.

—Masi

HOW TO HAVE SEXY, KISSABLE LIPS

With or without lipstick, the key is smooth, nonchapped lips. The easiest and quickest way to smooth out chapped lips is to use vitamin E capsules, which can be purchased from a drugstore or a health food store. The capsules are meant to be swallowed, but instead cut one open at night and apply the liquid to your lips (there will be more than enough—use the leftover liquid on your cuticles).

—DezG

HOW TO COVER UP A HICKEY

Don't just cover up a hickey . . . get rid of it! The trick is to really, really scrub it, as if you are trying to scrub it right off your skin. Then either wash your face with warm water or hop in a warm shower and give it a really good rub.

—blueintrinsic

HOW TO AVOID EYE INFECTIONS

Don't rub your eyes. I read somewhere that your hands/fingers are germy. As a person with a nervous habit of rubbing my eyes, it took me two bouts of pinkeye and a puffy right eye to finally get it through my head to stop.

—*hummer*

HOW TO KNOW WHAT SHAPE TO PLUCK YOUR EYEBROWS

If you've got thick eyebrows and you want to know what the plucked shape will look like, take a white eyeliner pencil and draw over the hairs you're going to take off—that will let you see what your brows are going to look like.

—*Gwendolen*

WHEN TO PLUCK YOUR EYEBROWS

Pluck before you go to bed, *not* before you go out.

—*Tamsen*

HOW TO REDUCE THE PAIN OF PLUCKING OR WAXING YOUR EYEBROWS

To minimize the ouch factor of tweezing your eyebrows, press a hot washcloth onto your eyebrows for a few minutes beforehand; the pain won't be as bad.

—*Hw92*

HOW TO HAVE GORGEOUS EYEBROWS

Don't pluck your eyebrows at the top; always pluck from the bottom of the eyebrow. It's usually best to get a professional to do them for you first and then you can just pluck the new hairs as they grow. Also, use strong bright light or daylight and a magnifying mirror. That way you can get all those hairs you don't normally see.

—waxy1086

You can tame rogue eyebrows for the day by spraying a little hairspray on an old toothbrush and then grooming them with that. (Trying to spray hairspray directly onto your eyebrows is a terrible idea for all sorts of reasons.)

—Twila

HOW TO MAINTAIN EYELASH CURLERS

The rubber on eyelash curlers cracks sometimes, and if you haven't noticed, it'll cut your eyelashes off. Turn the rubber around or buy a new one. They can be like a guillotine.

—Bridget

HOW TO HAVE A LONG-LASTING
CURL FOR YOUR EYELASHES

Heating your eyelash curler with a hair dryer first makes it far more effective. This is kind of like a mini-curling iron. Always test the heat of the curler on the back of your hand first, though. . . .

—Daphne

If you do not have an eyelash curler or do not like using one, then this is a tried and tested tip: Brush on the mascara, then, using your forefinger, hold the edge of your finger under your lashes and gently push up and hold until dry.

—kimberly1

HOW TO GET EYELASHES OUT OF YOUR EYES WITHOUT TOUCHING THEM

Just blow your nose with your eyes closed. Your eyes will water, washing out the eyelash.

 —*Weezy*

HOW TO IMMEDIATELY BRIGHTEN YOUR EYES

Using white or pale, pale blue eye shadow, dab a bit of shadow in a sideways "V" around the inner corner of each eye. Your eyes will look bright and wide awake. Shadow works better than liner or eye pencil as it is much subtler.

 —*CeeVee*

HOW TO GET FOOD OUT OF YOUR TEETH WHEN YOU'RE NOWHERE NEAR A TOOTHBRUSH

It may sound gross, but if you're stuck with nothing to use, the post or wire of an earring will work. You can clean it later in the bathroom, or use hand sanitizer on it before reinserting it in your earlobe.

 —*pmc1720*

Fold a piece of paper and use that as a toothpick.

 —*hschoi*

This is the *sole* benefit of being a smoker. . . . You can use the cellophane from a packet of cigarettes as emergency dental floss.

 —*Gam*

HOW TO CLEAR UP PIMPLES

Neosporin can be used for more than burns. If you apply Neosporin onto the whitehead or pimple at night, you will definitely see a change in the morning. Cross my heart.

—*shanequiacooper09*

HOW TO TAKE THE RED OUT OF A PIMPLE

Use lavender oil; it really does calm down the redness. Just a drop overnight will do the trick.

—*patstanley*

You can temporarily take the worst of the redness out of a spot with whitening eyedrops.

—*Olwen*

HOW TO PREVENT CROW'S-FEET

Always wear sunglasses on bright days to prevent squinting. Have your eyes tested regularly (yearly if you're over forty) for the same reason.

—*leggbarbara*

HOW TO STOP "AIRPLANE SKIN"

Pick up a free sample of a leading face mask at the beauty counter when you pass by (look for a colorless one). Samples are small enough to pass the airline restrictions, cheap, and easy to carry in your handbag. Clean and exfoliate your face before you leave your house; once you are in your seat, use a face wipe to clean off any airport grime and apply the face mask. Leave it on for the entire flight, drink a lot of water, wrap yourself up in a shawl to stay cozy, and get some sleep. Wipe off the face mask on arrival and you have had a great facial.

—*Amelia*

HOW TO MOISTURIZE AT A LOW COST

Lie in a very hot bath with a liberal application of extra-virgin olive oil on your face for thirty minutes and watch the lines vanish. This lasts only a few hours but is perfect for a night out.

   —higgy

My grandmother never used conventional moisturizer. Her remedy was this: Cut a large potato in half and rub it over your face and neck until the starchy moisture has dried; your face will feel a little bit crusty but not tight. Leave it on for five minutes, then rinse off with cool water.

   Her skin was magnificent up until she died at eighty years of age. I must confess I don't use the same method all the time, but I have used it often as it makes the skin feel very plump and refreshed.

   —Mandy

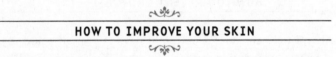

HOW TO IMPROVE YOUR SKIN

Apple cider vinegar smells awful, but it brings a radiant glow to your face. Don't use this when leaving the house or sleeping next to your man. But apply with a cotton ball when you can escape being sniffed out. I've also made a cleanser with honey, salt, and apple cider vinegar. Exfoliating, peeling, hydrating. Awesome.

   —vaportrailed

Wash your face with honey! Use pure honey (raw organic if you can get it)—just smooth a little on and rinse off. This can clear up acne and blackheads, and it's all natural. It's also antimicrobial and tastes good, too!

   —ZenMomma

HOW TO KEEP YOUR FACE LOOKING YOUNG AND SOFT

My grandmother is ninety-three years old and looks like she's barely seventy. She stayed out of the sun and put Vaseline on her face as a moisturizer every night for decades, and still does.

—KittenCarlisle

HOW TO CLEAN OUT CLOGGED PORES AND BLACKHEADS

Crush five or six aspirins with water to make a paste, leave on for about fifteen minutes, then rinse. Repeat twice a week.

—twigger

Make a paste using baking soda and a little water. It should be fairly thick but moist. Use the paste as a scrub to exfoliate clogged pores. Works like a charm!

—amandag

HOW TO MAKE YOUR OWN FACE MASK

I know it may sound crazy, but eggs are really good for making a face mask. Whip an egg white and then gently pat it onto the skin. Not only does it tighten and tone, but it also has softening properties.

—Lynz

· MAKEUP ·

OR HOW CAN IT TAKE SO LONG TO MAKE IT LOOK LIKE I'M NOT WEARING ANY?

STUCK in a rut? Been doing the same thing with the same colors for years in the belief that you know what suits you? Nothing is more aging. Applying makeup is *not* like shaving is for men. Our faces constantly change shape, color, and texture, and yet we cling to our old routines because with a new look we suddenly don't look like ourselves anymore. Well ladies, sometimes that is a good thing. The big cosmetic companies spend more than the annual GDP of some countries on developing products that actually work and make us more beautiful. Give them a chance. Whatever you're wearing, and whether you like your shoes or not, most evenings you'll be viewed across a table, so it's worth dressing up your expression instrument.

HOW TO ORGANIZE YOUR COSMETICS DRAWER

Attach a piece of elastic to the inside of one of your drawers with thumbtacks. You can then slot all your lipsticks and various small tubes behind it, and they will stop rolling around.

—*Jane*

Put a cutlery tray in your makeup drawer.

—*Magiwyn*

HOW TO FIND GOOD-QUALITY MAKEUP BRUSHES WITHOUT PAYING TOO MUCH FOR THEM

I go to the art-supply store. You can get different textures and sizes of brushes, and you can test them against your skin if you are sensitive.

I use a small rounded paintbrush to apply my foundation, and I have several different ones for concealer. You can even find an ultrathin one for eyeliner.

—*Masi*

HOW TO CLEAN MAKEUP BRUSHES

Use a gentle shampoo. Do not wash where the hair joins the handle; otherwise it will loosen the glue. After washing, take a towel and press out any excess water. Lie the brush flat on a surface such as a table, with the hair part of the brush exposed to air, so it can air-dry. It is crucial for the brush to dry thoroughly and in its shape. Don't wash your brushes more than once a month.

—*Replicant*

Add bicarbonate of soda to warm water and baby soap. Then rinse well and towel dry. The bicarbonate of soda helps to loosen and dissolve any stubborn grease and makeup, and removes any unwanted odors! Works wonders every time.

—*Kezabell*

HOW TO WASH MAKEUP SPONGES

Place your makeup sponges in the washing machine in the small net bags that detergent tablets come in.

—sgrimwade

HOW TO GET RID OF EYE MAKEUP

I have used baby oil for years. It gets rid of any mascara, it's very clean, and it doesn't dry the skin. Just put some on a tissue and wipe gently. However, if you want to reapply mascara immediately afterward, you need to wash off the baby oil first; otherwise you end up with big "Panda-eyes"!

—Anita123

Vaseline. It dissolves all mascaras (even waterproof), eyeliners, and eye shadows. Make sure it's warm so that it's soft and doesn't drag. Afterward make sure to wipe away all traces with a cotton ball.

—Nobodylikesasmartass

Olive oil does the same thing as Vaseline, but it's organic and not petrol-based.

—patriciao

HOW TO APPLY FALSE EYELASHES

Attach them to the base of the lashes that are already there, not to your skin.

—Magda

Stick down the inside corner first (use tweezers if necessary), hold it down patiently until it's dry, and then do the rest. Be careful not to get the glue in your eye (ow, ow). Don't try to stick the whole thing on at once; you'll end up in tears.

—Flapper

Let the glue almost dry so it's tacky before you put them on; if it's too wet, they will slide around.

—*Verity*

❧

HOW TO STOP MASCARA FROM SMEARING

Before applying mascara, lightly powder over the eye area using a brush and a loose neutral powder. This soaks up excess oil and helps thicken lashes.

—*leggbarbara*

❧

HOW TO APPLY BRONZER

Use a big brush and put it where the sun would hit your face—top of the cheekbones, brow bone, forehead, nose, and chin. The point is to look as if you're sun kissed, not colored in. And don't forget your collarbone.

—*Larissa*

❧

HOW TO MAKE LIPSTICK LAST LONGER

Apply liner and lip color as usual. Blot, then dab on a neutral pressed powder, followed by another layer of the lipstick. Blot again, and your favorite color will last for hours!

—*KellyM*

❧

HOW TO GET THE MOST OUT OF A TUBE OF LOTION

When you think your tube of lotion is finished, cut off the top and look inside. You will find you still have loads left. You can always use a clip to keep the top sealed.

—*waxy1086*

HOW TO CHOOSE THE RIGHT FOUNDATION

Test your foundation on your jawline, not your hand, to make sure it matches your facial skin tone.

—*Hw92*

Find the two shades that come closest, buy them both, and mix them at home every day. You'll be able to readjust the pigment level to match your natural color, which can change from day to day anyway.

—*Masi*

HOW TO TACKLE VERY DRY OR CHAPPED HANDS

Use foot lotion. I usually have really chapped, dry, and cracking hands, but I've found that cracked-heel lotions really work on smoothing them out. It's very thick and creamy, so it's good to use it at night or at least once a day. My hands look younger and my usually flaky palms, fingers, and cuticles look and feel almost normal now.

—*pjamas10*

HOW TO NOT GET LIPSTICK ON YOUR TEETH

After applying lipstick, wrap a tissue around your index finger, put your finger in your mouth and shut your mouth to blot the lipstick. Then smile.

—*noeleblue*

HOW TO PULL CLOTHES OVER YOUR HEAD
WITHOUT RUINING YOUR MAKEUP

If you need to pull clothes over your head and you've already done your makeup, put a large old pair of panties on your head so that they cover your face. They will protect your clothes and your makeup.

—Gam

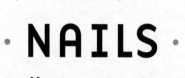

· NAILS ·

or How hard could it be to keep them looking nice? Very.

IT'S astounding how much effort many of us put into our nails, when a pair of nail clippers and a nail brush will do the job perfectly efficiently. And although you may not be conscious of it as you file away, the way you do your nails is a minutely small, terrifically specific, physical manifestation of a very conscious decision about how you want the world to see you. So small, that it is a matter of fractions of millimeters between our individual perceptions of "utterly chic" and "raging slut." I'm currently going for short with clear varnish, which I hope conveys (in the international language of Manicure) that I am practical, understated yet chic, and mindful of my appearance without being unduly obsessed with it. Last week it was very short and bright red, which I felt was excitingly contradictory.

HOW TO TAKE CARE OF A SNAGGLY NAIL
WITH NO EMERY BOARD

I always carry a matchbook in my purse. This way, I have matches if I need them and can also use the scratchy edge to file a nail if I can't find an emery board.

—*CeeVee*

HOW TO MAINTAIN A GREAT MANICURE

Keep a nail file in the car and one in your handbag. Basically everywhere, so one is always handy.

—*SamanthaCameron*

The thing that has helped me keep my manicure in perfect condition for up to two weeks is to apply a coat of clear top coat daily. This prevents the tips of your nails from chipping and they continue to look fresh.

—*blueeyes126*

HOW TO QUICKLY FIX A CHIPPED MANICURE

If you have somehow managed to chip your nail polish (as we all do . . . all the time), dip the affected nail into a capful of nail polish remover and pull it straight back out again. Let it dry (tip downward). This smoothes out the chipped end. Once it's dry, run your finger over it to make sure that it's smooth . . . if not, repeat. You can then paint straight over! Voilà!

—*sophie08*

HOW TO STOP BITING YOUR NAILS

These are a couple of ways I stopped:

First, I *always* had polish on my nails.

Second, I just thought about where my fingers had been, and what could possibly be under my fingernails. I don't think most people clean their nails before they bite them. I got grossed out by thinking about what could be under my nails. Skin cells, dirt, old food particles, etc. Yuck. Plus, I don't want my hands to look ugly anymore.

—*BodyEnvy*

HOW TO WHITEN NAILS

Use an old toothbrush and whitening toothpaste, preferably one of the slightly abrasive ones. Brush the paste gently under your nails and leave it on for a minute if you have time.

—*patsharp*

Get two bowls of warm water (large enough to soak a hand in) and add one of those fizzy denture-cleaning tablets to each bowl. Put a hand in each bowl and soak for at least fifteen minutes. Just as the denture cleaners work on stained false teeth, they whiten and brighten nails, too!

—*DezG*

HOW TO GROW HEALTHY AND LONG NAILS

Take folic acid supplements. After two years of constantly flaking nails, I've taken folic acid for three months and have strong, healthy nails again at last.

—*Cali*

HOW TO PAINT TOENAILS EASILY

To avoid being a contortionist, I have found the best way to paint my toenails is to sit on the stairs. My feet are instantly raised nearer to me on the steps below so that I can easily reach them and maintain my balance.

   —Linx

Paint those toes with wild abandon! Just do it in the evening so they can dry completely before you go to sleep. In the morning shower, any polish slopped on your skin will practically wipe away!

   —blazabla

HOW TO PERFECT A PEDICURE

Your toenails may look fab, but I'm betting your toes don't! Right before you get into the shower, dip a cotton swab into baby oil and run the swab over the cuticles, sides, and top of each toe. The heat of the shower helps the oil sink in and you'll emerge with perfectly varnished nails *and* healthy toes that don't look dry or scaly.

   —CeeVee

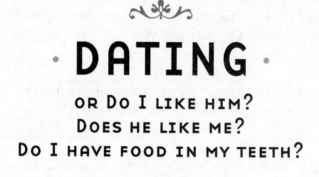

· DATING ·

or Do I like him?
Does he like me?
Do I have food in my teeth?

DATING is heaven or hell, depending on your attitude. Nowadays it is also a heaven or hell that you can experience at any age. You may still be doing it at eighty. However, as with makeup, you can get stuck in a rut. Developing your dating skills is just like flexing your muscles—get practical and proactive to keep up with the competition. Especially when there are so many ways to do it—from speed dating to Internet dating to old-fashioned being-set-up-by-friends dating. You'll never meet anyone at home on your own sofa, which is a very depressing thing to hear when you're feeling tired, inadequate, and low, but it's true. So get up and get out, so you can find someone to stay home with.

HOW TO MEET MEN

Avoid being the unapproachable princess in the tower. Smile and be able to stand alone for a while. No one is ever going to approach anyone in a big gaggle of girls.

—Helen

HOW TO TURN DOWN SOMEONE WHO IS ASKING YOU OUT WHEN YOU ARE NOT INTERESTED— WITHOUT LYING

Put yourself in the guy's shoes. Don't be cruel and don't burn any bridges. Someone whom you think you have nothing in common with today could be the man of your dreams in two years. People change. Always thank him for asking and tell him you are flattered, but . . .

- You're really busy these days.

- You're not sure the two of you have anything in common.

- Let's not do anything we'll both regret.

—Masi

HOW TO GET A GUY'S ATTENTION

The two things that a man likes about a woman are her mouth (whether or not she's smiling) and her eyes (whether she's making eye contact). I suggest you smile at him, sweetly and not in a creepy way. Also, try to maintain subtle eye contact, again not in a creepy way. Also, a laugh normally attracts male attention; if you laugh out loud at a joke, it shows that you're outgoing and fun, which men love. Try these things and I'm sure he'll be paying you all the attention you deserve.

—seksykt

HOW TO LET A MAN KNOW WHEN YOU LIKE HIM

If you've just spotted him, with solid eye contact and a smile
. . . if you've the courage!

—*hbkt83*

HOW TO CHECK IF YOU HAVE FOOD IN YOUR TEETH WITHOUT LEAVING THE TABLE

Discreetly use the blade of your knife as a mirror.

—*Emily*

HOW TO PREVENT OVEREATING ON A DATE

In my experience, men like women who aren't afraid of food. Eat
what you like! Good food is one of life's greatest pleasures, and if
he disapproves of your eating too much bread or going for dessert
on your first date, then he's going to make you miserable in the
long run.

—*Shepherdess*

HOW TO OFFER TO SPLIT THE BILL ON A DATE

What I always do is let the guy ask for the bill (this can sometimes take a while if he isn't assertive); when he gets it, say casu-
ally, "Right, what's the damage?" If he is going to split it with
you, he'll tell you how much; if he isn't, then he'll say that he's
paying; protest only once—"Not at all," or "Are you sure?"—and
leave it at that.

I'm not a money-grabber, but I usually have found that guys
who insist on paying on a first date are going to be better boyfriend
material than guys who are happy to split the bill.

—*star*

HOW TO KNOW FOR SURE IF HE LIKES YOU

I've definitely found that if a guy likes you, he will invariably find a way to tell you. If he's not interested, he won't make any special effort to speak to you or hang out with you. It really is that simple.

—*Nikkiwelch24*

HOW TO NOT SCARE MEN OFF

If a guy comes back to your house, there is nothing worse than a home that is decorated too girly. Toss the teddy bears; avoid lace. It only scares them.

—*Kendra*

HOW TO CONTACT A MAN AFTER A FIRST DATE

You should not be contacting him!

He should be the one doing all the chasing! However, if you haven't heard from him in three or four days, send him a text such as "Hey, just want to say thanks again for a lovely time on _____. We should do it again some time." If you do not hear from him within two or three days, move on. If he's not chasing you, then he's not worth bothering about—you can do better.

—*Lynz*

HOW TO STOP YOURSELF FROM CALLING HIM

What I do, though not always successfully, is change his name in my cell address book to "Don't" or something appropriate to whatever crime I feel he's committed, i.e., "inconsiderate bastard who canceled at the last minute."

—*annalouisa*

If you have his number programmed into your phone but haven't memorized it, write the number down on a piece of paper and then erase the number from your phone's memory. Next, place the piece of paper with his number on it in an envelope and seal it shut. On the outside of the envelope, write down all the reasons you don't want to/shouldn't call. It worked for me. Every time I read what I had wrote, I decided not to call.

—whitdb

Write an e-mail instead but do not send it . . . just get it out of your system.

—Sylviamuchnick

HOW TO KEEP HIM WANTING MORE OF YOU

Be gloriously happy and fun to be around. Laugh at his jokes. Crack your own. Goof off together. Tell him—sincerely—the little ways in which he's absolutely fabulous.

—zbandicoot

HOW TO BE A WOMAN MEN LOVE

9 THINGS EVERY MAN LOVES IN A WOMAN

1. She is an independent woman, not a clinger.
2. She is sexy and hot, but not slutty.
3. She remembers to do the little things, just like she did in the beginning.
4. She lets him pursue her.
5. She never utters the words "Where is this going?"
6. She imposes a two-drink maximum on herself when she goes out.

7. She never humiliates him in front of friends, family, or coworkers.

8. She watches her language.

9. She says yes.

   —*Textinthecity*

· RELATIONSHIPS ·

OR EVEN MY SHRINK SAYS
IT'S YOUR FAULT.

THERE'S this myth of the perfect man arriving on a white charger. Trouble is, when he eventually turns up, you're not sure the horse is the right color or size; or maybe it's got more teeth than you imagined. Aim for unconditional acceptance, and you might reach the happy medium between a woman's urge to change her man and accepting the fact that the only thing you can change about him is his tie. We all know that the most important relationship is with yourself. Whatever; why does everyone else seem to find this relationship thing such a breeze? News flash: They don't. They may just be better at keeping their own counsel. No one tells you how much work relationships are. Kind of like housecleaning, it's a case of constant vigilance and maintenance. And if you reach the conclusion that you've just got to get out, go back and read "Dating, or Do I like him? Does he like me? Do I have food in my teeth?" again.

"I think I fancy your dad" always seems to work.

> —*curlytops*

"I think you're the one; when I think about you, all I want to do is plan our wedding and imagine how darling our children will be." Never fails.

> —*sozo*

HOW TO BREAK UP IF YOU LIVE TOGETHER

I just asked my partner what he would do if he made me unhappy. He said he would leave, so I said, "I'm unhappy." He left.

> —*sandie*

HOW TO GET OVER A DIVORCE

Wake up. Get out of bed. Stay out of bed as much as you can. Clean your home of his belongings, but don't be mean. Box them up nicely, fold everything, etc. Put his stuff somewhere out of the way where you don't have to look at it. Give it time. Do all the things you want to do that you haven't been doing while married. Give it more time. And one day, when you wake up, the hurt won't be there anymore.

> —*Bookluvinmo*

HOW TO GET OVER HIM

Make a list of all the things you *don't* like about him (like forgetting your birthday, never calling when he said he would). Read it several times a day, and particularly if you're about to pick up the phone.

> —*Manhattanminx*

Delete all his texts, all his e-mails, and his number from your phone. Tell all your friends you don't want updates on how he's doing, and it will help you get over him quicker.

—Makenzie

No man is worth your tears, and the one who is won't make you cry!

—Louie

Be an actress. At first, getting over someone is a decision, not a feeling. The feeling of really being over him comes later, and in the meantime, if you run across him, imagine that you are Meryl Streep playing a part. Act indifferent. Polite but distracted. Eventually you'll get over him. There are lots more fish in the sea!

—asildem

HOW TO STOP YOURSELF GOING BACK TO YOUR EX

Write down as many bad things about your ex as possible; these can range from how badly he treated you to his weird bathroom habits or his addiction to sports—but the more, the merrier. Then take another sheet of paper and write down all your good qualities. This is a great thing to do with a girlfriend or a family member you're really close to. Let them encourage you to identify all those good points you aren't even aware of! Then sit back and compare the two lists. Who looks like the better package for a new relationship, you or him?

—Ladypenelope

HOW TO KNOW IF YOU'RE OVER HIM

If his number is still in your phone and at no point, no matter how drunk or lonely you feel, are you ever tempted to call or text him.

—Annabel

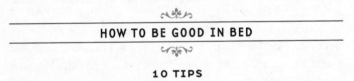

HOW TO MAKE A LONG-DISTANCE RELATIONSHIP WORK

Make sure you both want the same thing—a steady relationship. Take advantage of as many different methods of communication as you can—cards, letters, e-mail, phone, instant messaging, etc. Get cell phones from the same network so you can call each other for free, and then use them!

Plan your in-person visits for holidays, whenever possible. Use a webcam to "date" each other online and make the visual connection as well. It will take creativity and lots of communication, but it can be done.

—ImageCoach

My boyfriend and I had "movie/TV dates," where we would watch the same thing and be on the phone at the same time.

—Jrizzony

HOW TO BE GOOD IN BED

10 TIPS

1. Be hungry for it. Show some initiative, and take the lead.

2. Don't wait for him to tell you what to do. Go for trial and error. Experiment.

3. Make some noise. Show him you're enjoying yourself.

4. But don't scream like a porn star, unless that's what comes naturally.

5. Make sure your sheets are clean.

6. Swallow.

7. Ask him for what you want.

8. Let yourself go. He's not thinking about how fat your thighs are or how small your boobs may be. He's thanking God he's in this moment.

9. Learn to put on a condom with your mouth.

10. Vary your technique.

   —*buddha*

Be confident and enthusiastic. No one is just "good in bed." Everyone has insecure "off" days and partners that it just doesn't go smoothly with, but acting like you love sex—and more important, love your body—makes a big difference to how you feel about the sex you are having.

   —*benjizoot*

HOW TO GET HIM TO TALK MORE

My fella never talks—until I stop talking! Then I think he gets worried and starts asking me questions! Mission accomplished.

   —*Notwop*

HOW TO GET YOUR HUSBAND TO GO TO THERAPY

Tell your husband you need his help. Don't tell him you think there is anything wrong with him or that he needs therapy, or he'll surely dig in his heels. Few people will refuse to help someone in need. Once he's going, it will be up to the therapist to determine what your husband might need and how to get him to keep going. Having a male therapist who is older than your husband might help.

   —*sandrasimmons*

1. Try to find a male therapist, so he doesn't feel like you're ganging up on him.

2. Tell him why you think you need this (i.e., you need him to be on the same page as you).

3. If he won't go with you, leave the door open. You're going to do this; he's welcome to come.

   —*Midorable*

HOW TO FORGIVE HIM FOR PAYING FOR A LAP DANCE

I'm a lap dancer and can honestly say it is harmless fun. Some men have come in for dances, then a few minutes afterward say they're going home to give their other half a "good time." My point is that yes, they get turned on by the dancers, but it goes no further than that, and then their sexual thoughts return to their partner.

Most lap dancers have morals and do the job purely for money. I and my fellow dancers keep things strictly professional and the men respect that, too. He may have had a lap dance, but it's you he goes home to.

—*Missphant*

HOW TO GET OVER RESENTMENT

Remember what the great Carrie Fisher once said: "Resentment is like drinking poison and waiting for the other person to die."

Go ahead and be resentful for up to a day, just to indulge this very human feeling. Then make the conscious decision to get over it and move forward. Don't give the other person the power to make you miserable. That's like abdicating power over *your* one and only life.

—*CeeVee*

HOW TO KEEP YOUR RELATIONSHIP FROM BECOMING BORING AND STALE

Go out and do things that you wouldn't normally do, like taking a minicruise, playing hooky from work, wall climbing, car racing, anything, and do it spontaneously.

—*nicolet*

HOW TO KEEP THE ROMANCE ALIVE

Communication is key but can get lost in daily life. Make sure you take time out to reconnect by having a weekly date night. It doesn't need to be expensive or even romantic. Sometimes my sweetie and I just do the grocery shopping together. Just do something where you can talk to each other with no kids around.

—*sandrasimmons*

HOW TO KEEP YOUR SEX DRIVE ACTIVE WHEN YOU'RE STILL REALLY INTERESTED BUT JUST TOO TIRED IN THE EVENINGS, ETC.

Make plans to have sex—make it the best part of your day/week/month, whatever. . . . Talk about it, think about it, plan what you want to have happen. Sounds kind of weird, but it will help you get excited about it. Also, on nights when you don't feel in the mood, let him know, and let him try to find your mood for you. Sometimes having someone near and caring for you will arouse your sex drive when you don't expect it to.

Women are most often open to sexual intimacy when they feel close to their partner. Men feel close to their partners after having had sexual intimacy. Spending time with your partner sharing and exploring each other may help bring those feelings to the surface.

—*ramee151*

HOW TO MAKE YOURSELF HIS TOP PRIORITY

Be your own top priority. If you do not put yourself first, who will?

No one will ever look out for you better than *you.* Be your own worst critic—but also be your own best friend. Learn to be self-reliant so that you can survive—*thrive*—on your own, yet be equal in a partnership.

—*rachbu*

HOW TO KEEP YOUR BOYFRIEND INTERESTED

Make sure you are always the first to end telephone conversations.

—*Cali*

HOW TO MAKE HIM JEALOUS

Send yourself flowers with no card. They become a nonspecific threat.

—*Alessandra*

Make sure that when you are walking down the street you maintain eye contact with another man in a flirtatious way without your man seeing so that he carries on checking you out. Ideally walk a couple of steps ahead when doing this!

—*leylasadr*

HOW TO USE THE BATHROOM AT YOUR BOYFRIEND'S HOUSE DISCREETLY

1. Always go in after he's been, so he won't be going back too quick.

2. Go before a bath or a shower.

3. Matches and air freshener give the game away. You can hear the spray, and both have their own smell. I put the plug in the sink and run the hot water tap on full, then pour some hand soap into the stream—it all steams up and makes the bathroom smell like the soap! Which is how you'd expect it to smell, only stronger (though I doubt anyone will notice).

4. If it's evening, step 3 works even better with face wash because you use more of it and it usually smells more strongly anyway, plus it's your excuse for being in there longer.

Wow, I have put *way* too much thought into this.

—*Princess83*

HOW TO GET OVER YOUR BOYFRIEND'S
PAST RELATIONSHIPS

You have to remember that whatever happened before you came along, it is *you* who your boyfriend is with now. Do not worry or constantly wonder about what happened before—it will not make anything better or help you, and it will just annoy your boyfriend.

    —Lynz

HOW TO DECIDE TO TELL YOUR BOYFRIEND
THAT YOU CHEATED ON HIM

The only real rule in these situations is to treat others how you would wish to be treated yourself. If you do decide to tell him, you should give him as much respect and dignity as you can. (Try not to tell others who will gossip about it and make him feel foolish—he did nothing wrong.)

    —Wendy

HOW TO SPOT THE SIGNS OF
AN UNFAITHFUL PARTNER

- Receiving mysterious phone calls during which he answers only in monosyllables ("Mmm. Yes. No. Okay.").

- Arranging to meet up with friends and being coy about telling you where he's going, then not being reachable while he's out.

- Saying he's bought himself clothes (especially around his birthday or Christmas) or other items when he wouldn't normally.

- Buying new underwear (my ex actually had a pair of purple silk boxers—big alarm bells).

- Making more effort with his appearance.

- Visiting his mother more often, working overtime, going to the gym (yeah, right).
- Putting more miles on his car odometer than he should.

The other woman will do all she can, usually, to help the wife find out, so look out for perfume smells, lipstick marks, greeting cards he's hidden.

—*COLIYTYHE*

HOW TO KNOW IF HE IS "THE ONE"

- He understands.
- He tells you.
- He shows you.
- He listens to you.
- He's happy around you.
- He compliments you.
- He notices when you change something about your appearance.
- He takes care of you.
- His friends and family like you.
- He appreciates you.
- He asks for your opinion.

—*Textinthecity*

- Does he make you laugh and does he laugh at your jokes? A shared sense of humor is very important.
- Is he caring and helpful when you are ill?
- Is he tolerable when *he* is ill?

But if you have to ask those questions, he is possibly *not* the one! You should just know, I think.

—*operatix*

Focus his mind—by dumping him. If he is the right one, he will come and get you. If he is not, you have done the right thing.

—*Cheekster*

· WEDDINGS ·

OR I AM RELAXED.

THE proposal! The ring! The bliss! And then there's planning a wedding. It suddenly becomes all about what everyone else wants. Every family member will not only have an opinion, but most of them will turn that opinion into quite insistent advice. When it comes to weddings, *advice* takes on a whole new meaning. More like: "This is how I think you should have your dress/cake/ flowers/underwear/groom, and if you don't agree with me, I'll take it as a personal slight." Don't sweat the small stuff, just stay true to the top three things that are important to you. So if the napkins have to be coral because it's his mother's favorite color, get over it. And invite only the people who really mean something to you. Don't invite thousands of guests just so that you can have swans swimming around in the chocolate fountain.

HOW TO BUY AN ENGAGEMENT RING

When buying an engagement ring with your boyfriend, take him to a really expensive shop first; then he'll think the next place is a bargain.

—*Piper*

HOW TO GET LIVE CLASSICAL MUSIC AT YOUR WEDDING FOR A FRACTION OF THE COST OF PROFESSIONALS

Check with your local college. Most offer music courses. Choose advanced students who are looking to make extra money by performing at events.

—*Felicia*

HOW TO INCORPORATE YOUR FAVORITE CHARITY INTO YOUR WEDDING

Consider adding it to your list of registries.

—*koilyo1*

HOW TO SAVE MONEY ON WEDDING FLOWERS

Have the florist make arrangements that will be suitable for both the ceremony and the reception. This way they can be moved to the next location. Individual flowers can also be cut from church arrangements and reused as décor on the place settings.

—*Harmony*

You can use your bridesmaid's bouquets for table toppers at the reception and for the cake topper.

—*amycov*

HOW TO GIVE FLOWER GIRLS SOMETHING TO DO OTHER THAN THROW PETALS

For one of the weddings I recently participated in, the bride made "activity packs" for the child attendants to use during the ceremony and the reception. It included things like coloring books, crayons, picture books, stuffed animals, and little games. One of the flower girls made the bride a wedding card during the ceremony—it's one of her keepsakes now.

—*ramee151*

Bubbles are a great—and inexpensive—thing to add fun to a wedding, and it gives little bridespeople something to do when you come out of the service. They also look really cool in photos. Rice can be very painful when thrown!

—*LevantineLass*

HOW TO GET PEOPLE TALKING AT WEDDINGS

Write a quiz about the bride and groom (yourselves!) before the big day, with a range of questions that different people will be able to answer. On the day, have this and a pencil on the tables for people to complete when they are seated. This activity gets everyone talking to everyone to see who knows the answers. You can have a prize for the winning table, too!

—*Notnigella*

HOW TO GIVE THE PERFECT WEDDING GIFT

It's amazing how many couples look back on their special day and wish they had more pictures. Give the newlyweds a customized gift that they'll cherish forever. Take pictures at their wedding and create a coffee-table book with all the candid shots.

—*AdvocateForSmiles*

HOW TO MAKE PLANNING A WEDDING A HAPPY EXPERIENCE—THE ORGANIZED APPROACH

Make a draft timetable for the wedding and the reception. Include everything that must happen. Circulate it among relevant people. Get a consensus. Finalize the timetable.

Hire someone who's not involved to keep everyone—including all the staff as well as the bridal party—on schedule.

—*catinthehat*

HOW TO MAKE PLANNING A WEDDING A HAPPY EXPERIENCE—THE RELAXED APPROACH

Always bear in mind that planning a wedding can be a stressful exercise and that a wedding really is the most important day of most people's lives. Make every effort to be patient and tolerant of each other, even if everyone else seems to be getting touchy. You will all look back on the day with love and joy.

—*Cali*

· PREGNANCY AND PARENTING ·

OR I'M BEGINNING TO APPRECIATE MY MOTHER AFTER ALL.

THIS is the point at which you realize that you have been thoroughly lied to. No one tells you that when you are pregnant, your body image goes out the window and your ego gets trampled. No one tells you that your feet are going to become so swollen that you'll have to beg your husband to lend you his shoes. No one tells you that your age will also be your dress size. No one tells you that you will wear jewelry the size of walrus tusks, as you'll do anything to balance out the size of your belly. No one tells you that after nine idyllic months of being the center of attention, once you give birth, all people want to know is if you're back in your jeans yet. And yet . . . if anyone offered to take the little creature off your hands, you'd have to kill them before they got across the threshold. Welcome to the land of worry.

HOW TO PREVENT INDIGESTION DURING PREGNANCY

Ginger really worked for me—in any format—ginger biscuits, extract of ginger (found in health food shops), etc. Also pepper-mints.

—*Princessbella*

I ate a few fennel seeds (like $\frac{1}{2}$ teaspoon). It worked great for me and didn't feel medicinal.

—*mikcers*

HOW TO AVOID STRETCH MARKS

Find a stretch-mark lotion that suits you and get your partner to rub it in every night. It's fun, he's happy to do it (which means it will get done every night without fail or much prompting), and it gets him involved with the pregnancy. It also saves you the hassle of trying to reach over the bump and bend over, and you get a bit of a massage.

—*Amelia*

HOW TO DEAL WITH WATER RETENTION

Mix juniper essential oil with your body oil/moisturizer to get rid of water retention—this is amazing; my ankles halved in size.

—*Bridget*

HOW TO TURN OVER IN BED DURING THE LAST FEW WEEKS OF PREGNANCY

Buy a cheap satin chemise nightie, and you'll just slide and glide.

—*Billiedodd*

HOW TO REMEMBER WHICH BREAST
YOU NURSED FROM LAST

Remember which breast you last fed from by moving a bracelet from wrist to wrist. Really easy and really helpful . . . and a great excuse to buy yourself a pretty new bracelet.

—*Valerie*

HOW TO AID BREAST-FEEDING

Breast-feeding seriously dehydrates the mother's body, so drinking at least eight glasses of water a day is a must. Whole milk is also important because breast-feeding saps most of the mother's calcium supply and leaves her open to developing osteoporosis later in her life. The fat is needed because it is a healthy and essential supplement for the baby.

—*maryzeee*

During breast-feeding, drink as much fennel tea as you can to help with milk production.

—*LadyHelenTaylor*

HOW TO USE UP NIPPLE CREAM ONCE
YOU'VE STOPPED BREAST-FEEDING

As a lip balm! Works brilliantly!

—*LevantineLass*

HOW TO HEAL POSTPARTUM STITCHES FAST

Twice a day, sit in a tub of warm water with a few drops of lavender and tea tree oil. This stops infection, heals, and is great for soothing when the stitches get really itchy.

—*perky*

HOW TO PEE AFTER YOU'VE JUST GIVEN BIRTH

Peeing immediately after you've given birth is incredibly painful. As you pee, pour a cupful of warm water between your legs. It really helps.

 —*Marina*

This might sound silly. . . . Put Vaseline, just a touch of it, on the "torn" area before you pee. Part of what is so painful is the uric acids in the wounds—Vaseline will create a shield.

 —*yaylaliza*

HOW TO POO AFTER YOU HAVE JUST GIVEN BIRTH

Place your feet on two phone directories or something else that will raise your feet. It eases the pressure and makes the whole experience a little bit more bearable.

 —*ljp67*

HOW TO NOT FREAK OUT IF YOU'RE A FIRST-TIME MOM

Take what other mothers say with a pinch of salt. Bear in mind that many mothers lie to each other outright, and that mothers of other generations simply do not remember things correctly. So when your mother tells you that you were potty-trained at eight months, smile and thank her, and never give it another thought.

 —*LevantineLass*

The best advice I was given was from my mom: "Everything's a phase." It's gotten me through some dark moments as I try to bring up my twins!

 —*sparkles*

My advice would be to just go with it. Remember that babies are supposed to cry and puke all over you, and you're supposed to be completely exhausted most of the time. Make sure you get some fresh air every day—this is especially important in the beginning, when the days and nights roll into one! Oh, and make sure to meet up with your girlfriends regularly to keep yourself in touch with the real world!

—*ellenback*

HOW TO FEEL GREAT AFTER HAVING A BABY

Make half an hour a day for "you time." *You can find it!* Do your makeup, read a magazine, paint your nails, or do whatever else makes you feel great. And get dressed first thing in the day. This will motivate you to do something worthwhile with your day instead of sitting in your pajamas watching TV!

—*Vintageprincess*

HOW TO KEEP A POSTBIRTH MARRIAGE HAPPY

Don't forget the guy who was there in the first place. He may have gotten used to you putting him first—it can take a while for him to adjust.

—*Dorothy*

Your husband will be the one still around when your child leaves the nest, so it's worth making an investment in keeping him happy, too.

—*Amelia*

HOW TO KNOW WHEN IT'S "SAFE" TO HAVE SEX AGAIN

I have personal experience with sperm that lasted eight days (like the miracle of Hanukkah!), even though everything I've read says no more than seven. So you might want to avoid "relations" for at least nine days before ovulation. Theoretically the egg survives only a day or so after ovulation, so you should be able to resume three or four days later.

—serotonin

HOW TO GET A BABY TO STOP CRYING AND SLEEP

Put the baby down to sleep as usual and turn on the vacuum cleaner. This sounds weird—but it worked for my daughters.

—LondonMarian

HOW TO HANDLE BABIES WHO
ARE DIFFICULT TO BURP

I'm a nurse in a special-care baby unit; a lot of our babies are difficult to burp. This tip can be used by everyone! Place the baby on your knee facing away from you (this prevents any spit-up from getting on you). Supporting his head and neck and holding him firmly, slowly move the baby in a circle, without moving the legs. Think of it as if you were sitting on the edge of a bed and you moved the top half of your body in a full circle. It is important to do this gently, as you don't want any vomiting! Practice on a teddy bear or a doll first to get the idea.

—livliv

HOW TO BANISH THE PACIFIER

Santa took our two-and-a-half-year-old's pacifier. He took it for children who didn't have one and left an extraspecial present for a kind and generous boy. Santa collected the pacifier from under the pillow when he left presents. It worked *much* better than expected. We were dreading it. No tears at all.

—Clanger

We had "the pacifier fairy" visit us. We told our son what was going to happen a couple of days in advance, just to get him used to the idea that in two more nights, the pacifier fairy would be taking it to give to a baby. On "the night," he put his pacifier into a little basket and put it on the windowsill. In the morning, the pacifier fairy had left him a present as a thank-you. As I recall, he asked for his pacifier only twice after that and there were no tears or tantrums. I highly recommend it.

—wookiewoo

HOW TO KEEPS WIPES MOIST

I always store mine "facedown." The liquid that is in the wipes seeps to the bottom wipe, which is really the top wipe, and therefore when you turn the pack the right way up, the top wipe is moist and not dried out.

—anassa

HOW TO CURE CONSTIPATION IN BABIES

I find carrot juice a really good cure for constipation, even in babies. Just don't overdo it.

—Gretel

Prune juice works wonders quickly, too.

—sparkles

Straight apple juice; it doesn't take much, and babies like the sweet taste.

—asildem

HOW TO PREVENT DIAPER RASH

I use Vaseline on the baby's bottom as a barrier. It works well as it's waterproof and is also good for the baby's skin. Clean the baby's bottom as usual, then smear on a good amount and pop on a diaper as usual.

—*livliv*

HOW TO EASE DIAPER RASH

When changing a diaper, try drying the area thoroughly with a hair dryer on the cool setting.

—*Nigella*

HOW TO MAKE A TODDLER LAUGH

Admire and then ask if you can borrow their clothes. This never fails to elicit a laugh as they tell you raucously that you're *far* too big to borrow their clothes.

—*CeeVee*

HOW TO AVOID TANTRUMS

Best advice ever from my mother: *Never* ask a toddler a question to which he can answer *no*.

—*jennyfa*

Distract, distract, distract! If you know the telltale signs that a tantrum is coming, then distract your child by playing games such as I spy, etc. Or if you are shopping, include them—ask them to find which groceries you are looking for. Make everything into a game to keep them from getting bored.

—*LASHES*

My grandmother once told me of taking one of my cousins shopping. My cousin started to throw a tantrum, and my grandmother just stopped and said to the people around her, "Everyone, let's watch Kathryn throw a tantrum!" She said Kathryn quieted up in a hurry and she never had that problem with her again.

—sandrasimmons

I found with my kids that once a tantrum starts, we all leave the room except for the tantrum thrower. I also turn off the TV or any other distraction. Each time the child calls me back into the room, I calmly state that we will talk about it when they are calm. The first few times it can carry on for ages, but eventually you will be out of the room for only a minute before they are apologizing.

—Icemaideno504

If I was having a tantrum, my mom would say, "Don't laugh! Don't laugh!" over and over again. I'd collapse into fits of giggles every time.

—MaryPlain

To pull this one off, you really have to have no shame. When the child begins to throw a tantrum, simply lay down on the floor next to them and start screaming and crying. I've only ever had to do this once.

—dollymeh

HOW TO ENTERTAIN YOUR TODDLERS WHILE YOU GET DRESSED, DO YOUR MAKEUP/HAIR

Most toddlers love to stack and organize things. When I need some uninterrupted time to myself, I take out my special bag of hair rollers. Like most women, I have curlers of all shapes, colors, and sizes that I might not use often but would never get rid of. I make sure that there are no pins, clips, or anything dangerous, and I dump them all on the floor. The last time I did this, my kids spent almost an hour playing with them before they started to annoy me.

—*maryzeee*

HOW TO LEAVE YOUR CHILD HAPPY WHEN YOU LEAVE FOR WORK

I was a nanny for a number of years. The best thing to do is not just run out of the house but to prepare in advance. Make time in the morning so that you and your child can have special time together. Make sure to always remind her that you are leaving. "Remember, Mommy has to leave for work in ten minutes, but I will be back tonight." Make a very simple but very special routine every morning like getting up and getting ready, having breakfast, and reading a book together. If she knows that you have that time together, it will calm her down. Have a similar "special time" when you get home from work.

—*Melie*

Try getting the babysitter to divert his attention (with a DVD or a coloring book) after you have kissed him bye-bye. As hard as it is, try not to keep going back to reassure him once you have said good-bye, as this prolongs his tears and your sadness, too.

—*Joolz*

HOW TO KEEP YOUNG CHILDREN AND BABIES AMUSED ON LONG CAR TRIPS

Take some chalk and mark each child's first initial on one tire on the car. Every time you stop for gas, food, etc., see whose initial is closest to the ground. That person gets a prize. Sometimes we gave the winner $1 spending money for the trip, sometimes they got to sit in their preferred seat, and sometimes they got something from the "goodie bag."

—*sandrasimmons*

HOW TO AMUSE SMALL CHILDREN IN RESTAURANTS

Play the "what's missing" game. Each person takes a turn to remove something from the table while everyone else closes their eyes. When the item has been hidden beneath the table, the first person to realize what is missing is the winner. Just be careful that the bill isn't due. Once our poor waitress wondered why we appeared to be praying at the end of the meal. Even small kids love this game.

—*Steph*

Play the "a to z" game using a topic such as girls' names. Take turns thinking of as many as you can for each letter; at the end count up the number of passes each person has for when they couldn't think of an answer and went to the next letter. The person with the fewest passes wins.

—*Nicolamac99*

HOW TO END BICKERING AMONG SIBLINGS

This is one of my all-time favorite solutions. When the kids start bickering, tell them they need to sit and hold hands with each other for ten minutes. Just the *thought* of having to hold hands will usually stop the bickering—but if it doesn't, the actual *fact* of holding hands does the trick. Tell them if either of them squeals because the other is holding hands too hard, ten minutes are added to the punishment.

—*CeeVee*

If your children squabble about whose turn it is to take the front seat of the car, or whose turn it is to choose something first, you can solve this by writing each child's initials on the days of the calendar, alternating. Monday is child number one, Tuesday is child number two, Wednesday is back to child number one, Thursday is child number two, and so on for every day of the month. On the day that the child's initials are on the calendar, all day long she gets first choice on everything. If there's a disagreement, just say, "Whose day is it?" This completely solved squabbling for my kids for years.

—*asildem*

HOW TO CURTAIL NASTINESS BETWEEN SIBLINGS

If you are at your wit's end with siblings being nasty to each other, tell them the consequence is going to be purchasing and wearing a T-shirt printed with "I love my (sister or brother) (sibling's name)." Our son bought a shirt and we took it to a shop with an embroidery machine. His shirt said "I love my sister, Shelby!" and he wore it on several occasions (to school), much to his chagrin. The mere mention of the shirt has brought him around many times.

—*sandrasimmons*

HOW TO GET CHILDREN TO BEHAVE

We do a behavior star chart, and when the kids get a certain number of stars, they may get a treat. Also good is a time-out for bad behavior. They go to a special chair or sit on the stairs on their own to think about their behavior. I will never say, "You are" this or that, but, "Your behavior is" this or that. I believe in a lot of praise for everything; it's good for instilling confidence. The biggest gift we can give our children is confidence and self-esteem.

—*TaniaBryer*

❧

HOW TO GET CHILDREN TO BEHAVE IN PUBLIC PLACES

Be sure to always bring a bag of age-appropriate toys and books. Never expect young children to sit quietly in a public place. Keeping surprises handy in your purse is always a winner. At the grocery store, make shopping a game. Say "Help Mommy find . . ." and give them an age-appropriate item—something green or with the letter *L* or their favorite cereal. Engage them in the process.

—*krmrn*

❧

HOW TO GET KIDS TO SHARE

Getting kids to share toys is easy when you use a kitchen timer that pings! When it pings, it's time to pass the toy over.

—*Clanger*

The golden rule of sharing food between two children is one cuts, the other chooses.

—*Gam*

❧

HOW TO TEACH YOUR CHILDREN
TO PICK UP AFTER THEMSELVES

We tell our kids they don't need to worry about picking up after themselves, and that we're happy to do it. *But* (and this is a big "but") they're well aware that if *we* pick up something—toys, clothes, shoes—we have the option of giving it away or throwing it out. This generally keeps them in line and picking up after themselves.

—*CeeVee*

I had to use my allowance to buy back any toys/clothes/shoes I left lying around. I became tidy *and* thrifty!

—*CassandraM*

HOW TO DEAL WITH A BORED CHILD

For those long afternoons, have a "job jar." Fill it with folded slips of paper, each of which lists a chore or an activity. Have the child draw out a slip of paper and really follow through with making him do whatever's on the slip. Have a few fun ones in there, too!

—*asildem*

If they are under ten, get them to lie down on wall lining paper (very cheap per roll) and draw around their outline. Give them a box of crayons and tell them to draw themselves—full size.

—*patsharp*

HOW TO HELP YOUR CHILD DEAL WITH A BULLY

When my daughter was eight, a former friend of hers suddenly turned into a bully and gave my daughter no peace. There was nothing physical—just meanness and rudeness.

I told my daughter one thing bullies hate is cheerfulness and politeness. We practiced her responses to things the bully would say, which *really* helped—kind of like studying for a test, I guess. Pretending to be the bully, I'd say something rude to my daughter and my daughter would respond by being perky and cheerful. Our two favorite and most effective responses to anything the bully would say: "Thanks for letting me know!" *and* "Sorry you're feeling so crabby today!"

It worked *wonders* and drove the bully crazy enough that within two or three days, she started avoiding my daughter.

—*CeeVee*

HOW TO TEACH CHILDREN NOT TO GOSSIP

We tell our kids that if they feel the urge to gossip, they just need to ask themselves two simple questions:

1. Is it kind?

2. Is it true?

If they can't say "yes" to both questions, then they probably don't need to share whatever it is they want to say about another person.

We also tell them that they should picture someone saying the same thing about them—and how it would make them feel.

—*CeeVee*

HOW TO HELP CHILDREN THROUGH
THE FEAR OF GETTING SHOTS

You may laugh at this one, but it worked for me! Starting when my children were small enough to understand that shots can sting, I would tell them to hold on tight to my hand and I would let my bravery flow out of me and into them. It worked every time with all three of my children (two girls and one boy—now eighteen, seventeen, and fifteen).

—*sandrasimmons*

HOW TO GET A CHILD TO SWALLOW
A PILL WITHOUT GAGGING

Two ideas:

1. Have the child take it with something thick like pudding so she can't feel it as it goes down her throat.

2. Practice with Tic-Tacs.

—*Blueberrymuffin7*

HOW TO AVOID SUGARY CEREALS

Both of my children love healthy cereals, but when supermarket shopping they will ask for the sugary, fancy-packaged, free-toy-included types (of course!). For a treat I will sometimes buy what they want, but to avoid giving them a full bowl, I serve their normal cereal with just a sprinkling of the sugary/chocolaty one on top. They feel like they've had a big treat, and I'm happy because I know they've had their complex carbohydrate.

—*blueskye*

HOW TO GET CHILDREN TO EAT VEGETABLES

Try growing your own veggies; even with a small garden or patio you can grow tomatoes or potatoes in pots, even carrots. We have a small veggie patch and have beans, carrots, and potatoes growing. Kids love to see the process of planting, watering, and harvesting, and the food tastes so much better.

—*COLIYTYHE*

I feed my kids raw veggies as snack food while they watch TV. They are so engrossed in watching that they will eat anything fed to them, especially if it's just before supper and they are getting hungry.

—*woozle*

HOW TO GET YOUR CHILDREN TO EAT FRUIT

If you freeze a banana, you can tell children it's a Popsicle.

—*Sadie*

If you freeze grapes, they become like delicious tiny Popsicles. Children adore them and grown-ups think they are pretty good, too. Plus you don't have to toss slimy grapes when they become overripe or bruised!

—*rosepink*

HOW TO GET A CHILD TO EAT

If he or she refuses to eat, don't make too much of a fuss; just take away their plate and don't give them anything else to eat until the next mealtime—no matter how much they whine.

    —Dacia

HOW TO BRUSH SAND OFF WET KIDS PAINLESSLY

Sprinkle on lots of cheap talc—the sand drops off and dressing is easy-peasy.

    —Clanger

HOW TO CLEAN UP AFTER A CHILDREN'S PAINTING SESSION

If you put a little dishwashing liquid into children's paints before they start, it makes it a lot easier to clean up. And it doesn't affect the paint at all.

    —Rosa

HOW TO KEEP TRACK OF ALL THOSE TINY BITS AND PIECES OF GAMES

Tape a resealable plastic bag to the inside lid of the box and keep all the little bits in there.

    —Willa

HOW TO INSTILL A LOVE OF MUSEUMS

Don't try to go through a whole museum in one day. Sensory overload will kick in, and you'll end up enjoying none of it.

First buy a guidebook. Then—over a coffee elsewhere—decide on one room or exhibit to visit. Go straight to that area/piece, enjoy it, and leave.

Repeat this another day, or even a few hours later, to see other parts of the museum collection.

—pgrier

HOW TO BE PREPARED FOR KIDS BEING SICK IN THE CAR

I keep a couple of empty ice cream tubs in my car; any plastic tubs with lids will do. If my young 'un is going to be sick, at least he can aim it into the tub. You then put the lid on and put it in a trash can next time you stop. Make sure you get the next one ready after, though! Keep some strong-smelling disinfectant in the trunk, too, along with some wipes to mop up any spills and to mask the smell.

—COLIYTYHE

HOW TO HELP YOUR KIDS LEARN TO READ

Get your kids to watch foreign films—more specifically, ones with subtitles. It will make your child want to keep up with the subtitles and movie, so he will be forced to learn to read faster or fall behind. That speed-reading will transfer from television to books. The film can be educational or not. Japanese anime is great—the movies are fun and amusing—but make sure the anime is appropriate for your child. Some anime is quite mature and graphic.

—hummer

HOW TO PREVENT HEAD LICE

When rinsing my son's hair after it's been shampooed, I put a couple of drops of tea tree oil in the rinsing water. He covers his eyes with swimming goggles. Although there have been a few instances of head lice in his school, so far, thankfully, he has remained clear.

—COLIYTYHE

HOW TO GET RID OF HEAD LICE

You should steam clean all beds, sofas, chairs, etc.—anywhere it is possible for the head to touch.

Separate the hair into thin layers. Dip cotton wool in paraffin and dab it on the roots of the hair. Leave it in for a day and rinse the next day. It will leave the hair a bit oily, but it kills anything living in there.

—Nats

HOW TO GET RELUCTANT CHILDREN TO ENJOY BATH TIME

When the small one refuses the freshly drawn warm bath, pick him up, cooing words of endearment, and carry him gently to the bathroom, then toss him in the tub, clothes and all. Problem is, after that my son nagged me for years to do it again.

—ladydigger

HOW TO GET YOUR TEENAGER TO COMMUNICATE

Talk to your teenagers while you're apparently absorbed in something else (cooking, ironing, sewing, driving, etc.). You'll get more information without eye contact.

—Gam

Go for a ride in a car, just the two of you. If you are sitting shoulder to shoulder and you are not making eye contact, it's very easy for the kids to open up.

Also, talk to him like an adult. Don't be judgmental. I work with teenagers and I get them to spill their guts fast, because they know I'll listen without judging. Also, tell them about things you did when you were younger, and not just the goody-two-shoes stuff, but the things that were fun at the time but turned out to be a bad idea. And don't lie about things like drugs. Just tell them it was a different time and you didn't have all the information you needed to make the best choice.

Teenagers respect honesty and vulnerability.

—Masi

If the teenager is a boy, feed him. If the teenager is a girl, take her shopping. No matter the sex of your teenager, make sure you have dinner together as a family as often as possible. Cooking, eating, and cleaning up together naturally makes the perfect climate for conversation.

—sandrasimmons

HOW TO DEAL WITH SAYING NO TO TEENAGERS

Explain why you are saying no and ask them to come up with a solution to every point. Also, a genius move is to allow them to stipulate a coming-home time—I found it was often earlier than the one I would have set.

—ladykingston

HOW TO STOP ARGUING WITH YOUR DAUGHTER

This isn't a tip, but my daughter and I used to drive each other crazy most of the time. She died, suddenly, when she was in her twenties, and now I can never forgive myself for not being more loving and less bad tempered with her, however maddening she might have been. So remember, life can be short and you should try to keep the peace at all times.

—operatix

HOW TO BE A POPULAR GODPARENT

If you have lots of godchildren, send them a present on your own birthday instead of theirs—that way you don't have lots to remember. They will get so many presents on their actual birthdays that yours will stand out.

—*LevantineLass*

Send your godchildren postcards whenever you go away on vacation or business. When you're little, it means a lot to get your own mail.

—*Gam*

HOW TO STRENGTHEN THE BOND YOU HAVE WITH YOUR HUSBAND AND KIDS

Once or twice a year, have a family retreat. This means go grocery shopping at the beginning of the weekend so you're well stocked for food. Then turn off the computer, don't leave the house, don't answer the phone, and spend the whole weekend together, *just family,* playing board games, playing cards, watching movies, and simply spending time together with no distractions. Kids *love* this, and it's really a wonderful way to pass a weekend.

—*CeeVee*

HOW TO HELP YOUR CHILDREN MAKE FRIENDS AT SCHOOL

Make an effort to get to know the other parents and try to set up outings or get-togethers that will include the maximum number of kids.

The more parties and activities you organize, the more chances your children have to make friends.

—*Masi*

HOW TO STOP FEELING GUILTY ALL THE TIME

You cannot be the best mom, best employee, best wife, and best woman. Not all together! Don't push too hard. Start being honest with yourself, pointing out what is making you feel guilty. Then write down what can be achieved and when. If something is not possible for this year, relax. That's life and many women are facing the same challenge.

—*rafaelpay*

· WORK ·

OR AND YOU
THOUGHT SCHOOL WAS
A MINEFIELD.

WHEN I was starting up toptipsforgirls.com, a very wise friend warned me not to expect my friends to get too excited about it. At first I was appalled, but she told me not to take it personally. It is very human to think, "If my friend is doing it, it can't be that great" about a project or job we would be hugely impressed by if a stranger was doing it. It's got something to do with projecting our own inadequacies or something. In fact, my friends have been enormously and unexpectedly kind, even feigning interest as I bang on about Top Tips for hours on end. But I never expect it; it's not as though I'm having a baby.

HOW TO STOP PROCRASTINATING

You only need to know three words to succeed: *Don't dabble—FOCUS!*

    —Melody

If you have one big task that you're finding hard to tackle, try to break it up into manageable chunks. Either commit to finishing a chunk at a time, or to spending a full hour working on the project—with no distractions. It is amazing how much I find I can get done in an hour if I stop messing around and checking my e-mails every five minutes.

    —Alice

HOW TO STOP YOUR MALE BOSS (OR ANYONE) FROM MAKING PASSES AT YOU

As he leers toward you, scrunch up your face, peer closely, and say, in a slightly repulsed way, "You've got something in your teeth" as if it's something really revolting. He should be embarrassed and slink away to remove it.

    —Labink

Make friends with his wife/partner/daughter/son.

    —leggbarbara

HOW TO GET A RAISE OR PROMOTION

When negotiating a salary, pay raise, or promotion, imagine you are doing it on someone else's behalf. It's amazing how coy even the most accomplished women get when asking for money.

    —Felicia

Almost the most important thing is timing. Don't do it when it suits you; do it when it suits your boss. Learn to read her moods. Don't ask when she is frantically busy or in trouble herself. The best time is when things are going well and she is feeling happy and confident about the future of the company.

    —Paula

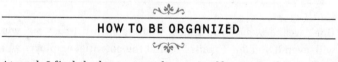

HOW TO MANAGE YOUR BOSS

Bring an agenda to every meeting—that way you can work through what you need, and not forget anything. Flatter and always give your boss credit without being a creep. If you make her look good, she will like you.

    —Trula

"Communicating up" helps. Always keep your boss informed (but briefly) with what's going on with your work. Don't assume she already knows this.

    Asking for regular reviews and welcoming feedback is another good idea. It engages your boss, makes her feel you want to succeed/improve, and keeps things from sneaking up on you (i.e., a problem that your boss sees and you had no idea bothers her).

    —bonviv89

HOW TO BE ORGANIZED

At work I find the best way to keep myself organized is to clear my desk before I begin another task. That way I won't get papers confused and I also have a larger space to work on. It makes a hell of a difference as you won't feel as bogged down. Clear desk . . . clear head!

    —sophie08

HOW TO SUCCEED IN BUSINESS

Never wound unless you can kill. It sounds brutal, but if you hurt someone badly, they'll remember. So don't wound unless you can completely take them out.

—*Callista*

HOW TO BUILD A RAPPORT WITH COLLEAGUES

Actually listen to what the other person is saying rather than focusing on your reaction to it.

—*Zoe*

HOW TO DRESS FOR A JOB INTERVIEW

Forget about wearing perfume. You may love it, but your future employer may not. Wear your makeup naturally. A smart pony-tail keeps your hair neat and is still professional. And under almost all circumstances, a suit is a must.

—*freemoniski*

HOW TO DO WELL IN A JOB INTERVIEW

Don't wear jewelry—you'll start fiddling with it (trust me, you will, even if you don't realize it) and the potential employer will get the impression that you are nervous. Also, when you first walk into the room, take a (subtle) sweeping glance around; that way you'll not feel inclined to stare at any objects and seem like a freak.

It seems obvious, but if you arrive ten minutes early, the employer can determine whether you're more likely to be early than late. Arrive more than ten minutes early and you may seem desperate, and you'll have been sitting in Reception being bored, so when you go in for "the kill" you'll have a bored expression on your face, won't be as fresh as you first were, and will probably have an annoying song stuck in your head!

Dress for where you want to be, not for where you are!!
    —*Mademoisellepamela*

Dress in comfortable clothes
(a touch of red is good for confidence).

Don't try to use words you're not familiar
with, in order to impress.

Don't change your speaking style.

Know your audience.

Know your subject.

Be yourself.

And visualize ending to rapturous applause.

If you can't believe in yourself, why would anyone else?!
    —*nursey*

※

HOW TO FOLLOW UP AFTER AN INTERVIEW

Don't leave the interview without a timetable of when a decision will be made. Specifically ask if all candidates will be notified or just those moving to the next step. Ask how notification will be made, via phone or letter. Send a proper note of thanks and follow that up with a phone call if you do not hear anything.
    —*whitlo*

※

HOW TO GET PEOPLE TO DO WHAT YOU WANT AT WORK

Don't be dictatorial; use language like "Let's . . ." or "Shall we try . . ."
    —*Candace*

HOW TO STAY CALM FOR A BIG PRESENTATION

Making a speech or a big presentation can be scary, but embrace the adrenaline as a superpower that will help you reach great heights. Keep repeating to yourself the mantra "I'm not frightened; I'm excited." It will help you reframe the task as an enjoyable experience—and people who are having fun are much more inspiring and appealing.

Whatever you do, don't start with "I'm so scared/nervous." No one came to hear you say that—they don't care and it will make you look inept.

—*Queenie*

HOW TO AVOID GOING RED WHEN
GIVING A PRESENTATION

If you're prone to severe blushing when you give a presentation, write your notes on green paper, or use a green marker on white paper. It's the same premise as color-correcting foundation—green neutralizes the red. I heard this tip at a presentation course, and it seems to really work.

—*suejak*

HOW TO SET UP A HOME OFFICE

Try to keep it away from busy areas that will distract you, like the kitchen. Also make sure the TV is out of sight—lest it tempt you!

—*Tamsen*

Buy a bigger filing cabinet than you think you could possibly need. The more files you make, the easier it is to keep paperwork, etc. tidy.

—*operatix*

HOW TO LOOK COOL IN MEETINGS

If you want to give an impression of seriousness and influence, lean in to the table. Putting your elbows on the table (folded in front of you) also adds to that impression.

If you are in a meeting with vendors, lean back in your chair to give an impression of casualness—it helps in your negotiations.

A FEW THINGS *NOT* TO DO

1. Smile too often (though cool smiles are useful, moderate your natural instinct to oversmile)

2. Cross and uncross your legs (gives an impression of nervousness and draws attention to your legs—save it for the hot date!)

3. Play with your hair

4. Sit with your hands in your lap (hidden hands imply hidden plans—and it makes you look meek).

   —*citygrrl*

HOW TO MAKE BETTER TIPS AS A WAITRESS

I read an article while I was waitressing in college that suggested when taking an order, try to be at eye level of the customer. I worked in a fairly casual restaurant so I would just squat down when taking an order. It also said to try to personalize the service whenever possible; writing "Thank you" and your name on the check would be an example. I did find that the eye-level thing really seemed to work and increase my tips.

   —*Lilacs*

HOW TO REGAIN CONTROL OF YOUR
TIME FROM E-MAIL, ETC.

Pick just a single time each day when you have X amount of time free—say, thirty minutes or an hour—really, whatever works for you. Then use this time period and *only* this time period to check your e-mail and return phone messages. You'll find that it makes you more focused and more attuned to your own personal priorities. Using this approach also takes far less time than checking both regularly throughout the day.

　—*CeeVee*

HOW TO CLEAN YOUR COMPUTER

First make sure everything is disconnected, then using a microfiber cloth dampened with a white vinegar/water solution and squeezed out well, wipe over. For grimy keyboard keys, a cotton swab moistened with the same mixture, then squeezed out into the microfiber to avoid drips, will get the job done. Do not fear that the vinegar smell will prevail, as it is gone within seconds and takes nasty smells like cigarettes with it.

　—*PoshPaws*

Vacuum over the keys with the nozzle, to get rid of dust and bits between keys. Wipe the rest with a moist wipe.

　—*girlies*

HOW TO DEAL WITH A DIFFICULT,
OLDER, INSECURE FEMALE BOSS

Compliment her clothes, accessories, etc. Get her talking about herself more. Make her feel really interesting and as though you are looking up to her—in awe almost! Ask her for advice about things that you may already know the answer to, which will make her feel superior and in control. It may be difficult initially, but she will begin to trust in you and you may end up enjoying her company!

—*whiskas*

HOW TO DEAL WITH A COLLEAGUE WHO IGNORES YOU

This person is threatened by you. This is usually why someone is extremely rude or ignores a coworker, unless they have a defective personality. Take comfort in the fact that you have something that your ill-mannered coworker wants, e.g., the approval of a higher-up, knowledge, clothes, good looks, etc. The only way to handle a person such as this is to kill them with kindness, especially when your superiors are nearby. It is so much fun to make the other squirm when they have to be nice!

—*byronspsbatt*

HOW TO DEAL WITH AN ANNOYING COWORKER

Keep focused on the fact that if you find him or her annoying, it's highly likely that many others do, too. Keep evidence of your annoyance very subtle—with a slight frown—while being overly patient and kind. And look out for how many times you catch a sympathetic eye across the room.

—*Meredith*

Understand that wherever you go in life, and whatever you do, you will be confronted with those who seem to be in this world only to make your life more difficult. The high road is more scenic but overrated.

Stealing all of the annoying coworker's staples, paper clips, and pens or "rearranging" things in his or her office space can be a harmless way to make those annoying ways more bearable.

—*citytimes*

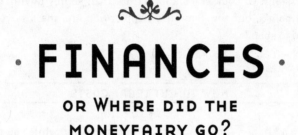

· FINANCES ·

OR WHERE DID THE MONEYFAIRY GO?

WHILE you, dear reader, are probably a financial wizard, many women reading this book will suffer from Money Fear. It's not as though they aren't capable, intelligent women, and this isn't about some kind of financial incontinence that leads to bankruptcy. It's just an intense boredom bordering on narcolepsy when it comes to financial matters, which leads to not making the effort to understand what's going on, which leads to a reluctance to open bank statements, which leads to more ignorance. And we all know that ignorance breeds fear. The only advice I can give is: Don't assume that a knight with a shining calculator will one day arrive to slay that financial dragon for you—just tackle that accounting head on.

HOW TO AVOID IMPULSE BUYING

Get happy. Of course, it's a lot harder than simply buying new nail polish, but the genuinely happier you are, the less you'll need to spend.

—*JCF*

HOW TO CUT LEGAL COSTS

Keep a kitchen timer on the table in front of you while you talk to your lawyer, even when you go to his office.

—*Magda*

HOW TO GET THE MOST BACK FROM YOUR DEPOSIT ON A RENTED PROPERTY

My partner photographed all the defects in his apartment on the day he moved in, had the pictures developed in an hour, and then sent the photos to himself via certified mail. When he received them, he left them unopened. When it came time for him to leave, he had photographic evidence of all the problems, and the postmark on the envelopes proved that they were there on the day he moved in and weren't his fault.

—*blonde36er*

HOW TO CUT DOWN ON BILLS

Use the dishwasher, washing machine, and dryer at night. I have heard the rates are cheaper. I tried it, and my bill was $20 less for that month.

—*pbales7349*

Make your own coffee/tea instead of pumping Starbucks' wallet.

Walk or bike instead of driving or taking public transportation. Save yourself gym and transportation bills.

—*vaportrailed*

Bring lunch to work with you—you can save hundreds a month; also it's generally healthier.

—*cleopatra11*

꧁⚜꧂

HOW TO SAVE MONEY WHEN SHOPPING

꧁⚜꧂

Put a little notebook in your purse. Before you impulse purchase a nonnecessity, write in your notebook what it is, where it is, and how much it is. If you're still thinking about it a week later and can afford it, go back and purchase it. Allow yourself only one notebook purchase a week. Chances are you'll either lose your enthusiasm for the item or find something you want more. Plus it just might be on sale when you return.

—*CreativeRiddle*

Ask yourself, "Do I really need it?" Realize that there is a difference between a need and a want. You should fulfill your needs but not always the wants.

—*Belalove*

꧁⚜꧂

HOW TO SAVE MONEY WHEN GROCERY SHOPPING

꧁⚜꧂

Put grocery shopping off for a day or two. Sometimes I am tempted to go shopping before I really need to. If I wait a couple of days, I have to get a bit creative with leftovers and existing food. Once you have a fridge full of new groceries, the older ones are less likely to get used. I try to use up all my fruit and veggies before making another trip. Stir-fries are a good way to use up veggies, and it is easy to invent new pasta salads using dressings and the last few tomatoes, etc.

This eliminates an entire grocery trip each month and makes me use what I have bought already. I would have to clip a lot of coupons to save this much!

—*Melaniezelanie*

HOW TO PAINLESSLY SAVE MONEY

Have a direct debit that comes out of your account into a separate savings account on the day you get paid. You won't even notice it's gone, as you are already feeling flush.

—*Vintageprincess*

I keep all my receipts from daily purchases and make a point to log it onto my weekly spending spreadsheet at the end of the day. The more you spend, the worse it makes you feel at the end of the day recording it all. Now, at the end of each week I always have something left to save.

—*chantlove*

HOW TO SAFELY DISPOSE OF RECEIPTS

To dispose of small items like receipts showing your bank card details when you don't have a shredder, simply keep a container of water to pop them in, leave them to dissolve thoroughly, then throw them away.

—*ladydigger*

We keep a jar and everyone puts their spare change in it. When it fills up, it's time for my two daughters and me to have a Girls' Day. We take the change to a coin machine and get some cash and then we vote on what to do. We've done this all throughout my girls' childhoods and it's become a great family tradition. Even my son and husband contribute their change, and on more than one occasion my husband has added some "bills" to give us a bigger budget.

—*sandrasimmons*

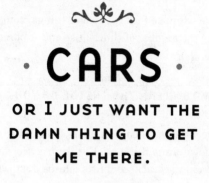

· CARS ·

OR I JUST WANT THE DAMN THING TO GET ME THERE.

A great truism is that every single motorist (male or female) believes that anyone who drives faster than him or her is a maniac, and anyone who drives slower is a moron. But the difference between the sexes is that when overtaken, many men can barely suppress their primal urge to race, while we find it impossibly hard not to suck our teeth and mutter, "Lunatic." Cars also divide the sexes in the most unexpected way: Women, commonly acknowledged to be the far more emotional gender, can be quite ruthless and cold when it comes to their cars, whereas men can get all anthropomorphic over a pile of rusty metal on wheels. And yet they appear immune to puppies and kittens. It's a wonder we manage to continue the human race with differences like that.

HOW TO RETRIEVE THINGS THAT SLIP
DOWN THE SIDES OF CAR SEATS

I always have a fondue fork to retrieve things from tight places.
It is amazing the number of times I use one at home, too.

—*MaryEllen*

HOW TO CLEAN THE INSIDE OF YOUR CAR

To clean the hard-to-reach places, like the joins in the dash-
board and down around the stick shift, use a clean, dry paintbrush; it gets in the cracks and lifts out the dust, which you can
then wipe away.

—*Tatchull*

HOW TO GET YOUR CAR OUT WHEN YOU'RE
STUCK IN THE MUD OR SNOW

First try putting sticks, branches, or the floor mats under the
tires for traction. If that doesn't work, try letting a tiny bit of air
out of your tires.

—*Queenie*

Keeping a bag of kitty litter in the trunk of the car in the winter
helps with this. Not only does the extra weight help, but kitty litter will give the car some traction on ice or in mud.

—*suejak*

HOW TO NOT PAY TOO MUCH FOR A CAR

1. Do your research on the Internet and figure out how much
   the invoice price for your car with all the options should be.
   Websites will also list a manufacturer suggested retail
   price (MSRP), as well as the market price most people are
   paying (falling between the invoice price and the MSRP).

2. Also look up any dealer incentives that are currently being offered by the manufacturer. The incentives will bring down the invoice price you previously found.

3. Now that you have your highest price (MSRP), your lowest price (invoice), and the reasonable price (market), call up dealers and play them off of each other in an attempt to drive the amount you pay as close to the invoice price as possible. For the first dealer you call, right off the bat tell them about all the info you found. ("Hi, I'm interested in your model XXX, for which I found the manufacturer is giving you a dealer incentive of $$. My own research quotes the fair market price as $$, so minus the dealer incentive, $$. I'm shopping around and would like to know what is the best offer you can give me on this car.") When you lay your cards out, the dealer knows you are an educated consumer. If you are going into the dealership in person, bring printouts of the webpage.

4. Once you have an initial offer from several dealers, call back the dealer with the lowest offer.

   —*at204*

HOW TO SAVE MONEY ON GAS

If you've turned your car into a giant storage bin and endlessly cart all sorts of junk around, clear it out! A heavier car uses more gas.

   —*Autumn*

HOW TO FIND YOUR CAR AGAIN AFTER PARKING IN A LARGE PARKING LOT

Tie a colored ribbon around the top of the car antennae. You can spot the ribbon a good distance from the car.

   —*Midge*

HOW TO FIND YOUR CAR AGAIN AFTER PARKING

When you are parking in an unfamiliar area, use the camera on your phone to take a picture of the nearest street sign.

—*neets22*

HOW TO MAKE YOUR CAR SMELL FRESH

I put dryer sheets under the seats. They smell great. Replace once a week.

—*0002mcl*

HOW TO AVOID STATIC SHOCK
FROM THE CAR AFTER DRIVING

Before you get out of the car, touch the door frame and then step out; keep touching the metal while you put your feet on the ground. The electricity will be discharged.

—*JuliaM*

HOW TO CHECK TIRE PRESSURE

To avoid getting your hands dirty, always keep a pair of disposable gloves in your car glove box for when you need to check your car's tire pressure.

—*sallyl*

HOW TO CLEAN OIL OFF A DRIVEWAY

If the oil spill is new, cat litter will absorb it. Just sprinkle enough to cover the oil stain, let it sit for a few days, and then sweep up the mess.

—*ramee151*

Cola works. Simply pour it on the stain, leave it for about an hour, and wash it off with very hot water and a stiff brush.

—*asherlox*

HOW TO REMOVE DENTS IN YOUR CAR

Before you admit to denting the car, try pulling a small dent out of the bodywork with a toilet plunger.

—*Karen*

· GREEN TIPS ·

OR FAT KEEPS YOU WARM, THEREFORE ENERGY SAVED, THEREFORE PLANET SAVED. NOW WHERE ARE THOSE CUPCAKES?

CLIMATE change, anyone? Whether you believe in it or not, the benefits of at least cutting down on waste of any kind are indisputable. The trouble is, rather like going for a mind-shatteringly exhausting workout, the beneficial consequences of our good intentions and even painful actions are incredibly hard to see. And not only are they hard to see, but we are going to have to learn to love the mild feelings of deprivation that so often accompany eco-logically sound resolutions—just as we convince ourselves that those screamingly stiff muscles are, contrary to all physical sensation, a good thing, and represent a future in which we are blessed with Elle Macpherson's bottom.

HOW TO SAVE WATER

Rather than putting bricks in your toilet cistern so that it uses less water (as they can begin to disintegrate and block your drain), it is better to fill a couple of small plastic bottles with water and drop them in.

—*keikei*

Invest in a water barrel in your garden. You can catch rainwater to use on your plants without depleting your water supply. Plus it has all sorts of minerals and nutrients in it. The barrels don't cost a lot, but are very effective.

—*nikkiwelch24*

This may sound weird, but in the winter I have a hot water bottle most nights. In the morning I use the old water to water my house/garden plants.

You can also use water from boiling pasta or vegetables once cooled to simply tip on your garden.

—*smithers33*

Wash fruit and vegetables in a small bowl rather than under a running faucet.

—*Annewayman*

If you turn off the faucet while you're brushing your teeth, you'll save about 2 gallons each time. And take a shower instead of a bath; that will save about 15 gallons.

—*Rhea*

HOW TO TELL IF YOUR HOUSE
IS PROPERLY INSULATED

If your roof still has ice on it when those all around you have lost theirs, your roof isn't loosing heat like the others are.

—*zoogirl*

HOW TO CHECK YOUR FRIDGE SEAL EFFICIENCY

To check the seal on your fridge door and make sure you're not wasting electricity, slide a dollar bill into the door seal. If it falls out, replace the seal or get a new fridge.

—*Tooke*

HOW TO SAVE ELECTRICITY

Amazingly, your freezer and fridge use much more electricity if there isn't much in them, so keep them as full as you can. And you should defrost your freezer regularly so that it works efficiently.

—*Marina*

If you go away in winter, you can turn your thermostat right down to only 41 degrees F—this is still warm enough to prevent pipes from freezing and bursting.

—*Wanda*

HOW TO REMOVE MAKEUP WHILE SAVING THE PLANET AND YOUR WALLET

Instead of using cotton or tissues to remove makeup, keep a muslin cloth in the bathroom and use that. The superthin ones dry super quickly.

—*LevantineLass*

HOW TO RECYCLE MAGAZINES

Bring them to the gym/doctor's office/any other waiting area and leave them for others. Also, consider getting alternate subscriptions with a close friend; read then trade.

—*DanielleDC*

HOW TO MAKE YOUR HOUSE "GREENER"

Unplug everything that you don't use on a daily basis, like a VCR or DVD player. Try to keep everything electric that you do use on a daily basis either plugged into a power strip that you can easily just switch off or in a place where it's easy to unplug. Try to make it a daily routine to unplug electrical items before leaving for work/school. Electrical items still draw power, even if they're not on!! It may even save money on your power bill.

—*Sweetie1027*

I ensure that my central heating is more efficient by having my curtains lined to retain heat in a room. My heating is only on twice, for short periods, during the day/night, when I'm actually in my house, and to ward off condensation/mold. Otherwise I just put on another layer. I burn candles when watching TV/listening to music (nice ambience and less electricity). I turn off all my lights, except in the room I'm in. I never boil more water than I need for a cup of tea/coffee. I try to use natural cleaning products (vinegar, bicarbonate of soda, lemon juice) instead of chemicals.

—*Nikkiwelch24*

HOW TO RECYCLE JUNK MAIL

I shred it all and add it to my compost bin, which will eventually make my plants grow.

—*Redlady*

HOW TO CUT DOWN ON PRODUCT WRAPPING

Unwrap everything you can in the store and leave it there. Maybe someday the retailers will force manufacturers to cut down on useless wrapping.

—*Cali*

· HOLIDAYS AND GIFTS ·

OR I CAN'T BUY YOU LOVE, LONG LIFE, OR HAPPINESS . . . SO WILL A SCARF TIDE YOU OVER?

IF there's one certainty after death and taxes, it's that many of us will be genuinely surprised—nay, amazed—by the arrival of the holidays. Normal, intelligent women who are great at planning their careers, their budgets, and their children's social lives often seem baffled by a herd of family members who are expecting to be fed turkey with thirteen side dishes and be given sundry items wrapped in brightly colored paper with chic yet festive trimmings. Extraordinary that we, the proudly self-proclaimed multitasking gender, who can simultaneously talk on the phone, send an e-mail, curl our hair, and make lunch, find it impossible to hold in our heads that December will need to be planned for.

HOW TO WRAP PRESENTS FOR YOUNG CHILDREN

Use aluminium foil.

—*mrsL*

Use the colored funnies section from the Sunday paper.

—*vampriss666*

WHAT TO DO WITH OLD CHRISTMAS CARDS

Cut around the pretty bit of a card (pinking shears are ideal) either in a square, round, or oblong shape; punch a hole at the top and thread with pretty ribbon; and use as parcel labels. Make sure there's no writing on the other side!

—*waynetta*

HOW TO DECORATE THE TABLE

Forget a fancy flower centerpiece (they don't last in centrally heated rooms); just pile clementines (with leaves attached, preferably), fir cones, and shiny baubles on a dish or a plate.

—*waynetta*

Wired ribbons cut into the appropriate length and fastened with a drop of glue make wonderful, festive napkin rings.

—*Ilana*

HOW TO STORE DELICATE DECORATIONS

If you have one of those sock-drawer dividers, it will work just as well in a cardboard box to keep your baubles separated and safe. Also, if you get the polystyrene apple trays, these work, too.

—*Theresa*

HOW TO STORE CHRISTMAS-TREE LIGHTS

Roll up a thick newspaper and tape it into a tube, then wind the lights around it. When you're ready to decorate, simply unwind and there are no tangles. You can use any cardboard tube container as well.

—*Judi*

HOW TO DECORATE ON THE CHEAP FOR THE HOLIDAYS

This is cheap, cheap, cheap and looks chic, chic, chic. Fill whatever clear containers you like (vases or anything else) with white rice and/or cranberries (they look nice separately or mixed together). Put white candles in the cranberries and red candles in the rice. It's an easy way to incorporate Christmas colors into the house, and it looks nice for a couple of weeks before you have to chuck the cranberries.

—*CeeVee*

Got spare lights? Get out your clear vases and fill them with the lights. Arrange the vases on top of a surface where you can plug in the lights without the cord going across the floor, such as on top of the TV cabinet.

—*Jillaroo95*

HOW TO ENHANCE PLACE MATS, ETC. AT CHRISTMAS

Decide on the color you want for your Christmas table that corresponds with your décor and tree; then choose shiny good-quality wrapping paper and wrap it around your place mats, dinner mats, etc. . . . Your table will look colorful and Christmassy!

—*gillybags1*

HOW TO CREATE HEIRLOOM ORNAMENTS

Have simple silver ornaments engraved with the names of family members and pets. When someone passes away, their ornament is hung at the top of the tree, "close to heaven." When a new pet arrives, or a baby is born, have a new ornament engraved. When children go off on their own, they take their ornament with them to hang on their own first tree. Every year it is meaningful when my children hang Grandma's ornament "up near heaven."

—*asildem*

HOW TO STOP OVEREATING DURING THE HOLIDAYS

To stop yourself from overeating at Christmas or Thanksgiving, simply tie a piece of string around your waist before the meal—under your clothes. It shouldn't be too tight; you should be able to get a fist between it and you. When it starts to draw blood, you should probably stop eating.

—*Minerva*

HOW TO BE PREPARED FOR EVERY SPECIAL OCCASION

Buy birthday, Christmas, engagement, and baby cards as you see them, so you're ready for every occasion.

—*Alice*

HOW TO BRING A GREAT HOUSEGUEST PRESENT

Instead of flowers or chocolate, take a bundle of new good books when you go to stay with someone. A selection of the latest bestsellers is always welcome. Also, a selection of hard-to-find magazines, especially if you are going to the country, makes a good present.

—*LevantineLass*

WHAT TO DO WHEN A HOSTESS GIFT IS RETURNED TO YOU BY THE HOSTESS HERSELF

Give it back to her the next time you visit, and see how many times the gift goes back and forth before you both admit you'd have preferred a bottle of gin.

—*pgrier*

HOW TO RECYCLE GIFTS

When you receive a gift you don't want and you want to save it to give to someone else, remember to store it with a note to say who it was from so you don't end up giving it back to them!

—*button*

HOW TO CREATE THE PERFECT GIFT FOR VERY CLOSE FRIENDS

For a perfect gift for a momentous occasion, simply buy a photo album and on a double page place one picture of another friend; on the opposite page, have that friend write a personal message for the recipient. Then just place other cool pics in the rest of the book! Decorate to finish!

It's great if you have a group of close friends; this is a perfect gift for eighteenth birthdays.

—*seksykt*

HOW TO GIVE FOR A SPECIAL OCCASION

To make a milestone birthday (like a thirtieth or fortieth) even more memorable, plan ahead and buy thirty (or whatever number) small gifts, wrap each individually, and give one per day for each of the thirty (forty, fifty . . .) days leading up to that birthday. Soap, candy, inexpensive earrings, etc. are great ideas, and the recipient gets to celebrate in advance of the big day. Smiles all around!

—*lnmop*

HOW TO BUY THE PERFECT GIFT

If you're unsure of what to get, get a large gift bag and buy lots of small gifts that you know will come in handy and prevent the person from having to purchase items they normally use (i.e., magazines, a certain face wash, lip gloss, etc.). Just think how much you'd love it!!

—*Kirsten*

Don't buy gifts at the last minute. If you see something your partner or friend might like a month in advance, buy it!

—*Anita123*

HOW TO SEND GREAT FLOWERS

Request that the arrangement be composed of a single type of flower, in a uniform color. This guarantees against ragged, cheap-looking arrangements from a remote florist.

Even an arrangement of all daisies or carnations looks better than a similarly priced "spring bouquet," which is florist code for leftover alstroemeria and fern leaves shoved into a basket.

—*fashionvictim*

HOW TO TIE A PERFECT BOW

When you're tying the actual bow bit, take your lace or whatever over first, rather than under, and your bow will be straight.

—*thepoet*

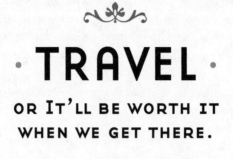

· TRAVEL ·

OR IT'LL BE WORTH IT
WHEN WE GET THERE.

THE rush to relax can cause travel-induced hysteria. I wonder how many of you have been in such a frenzy to kick back that the first two hours on the sun lounger have nearly required CPR? We are all so used to achieving in our working lives that we feel we have to vacation as successfully. The goal of many holidays is now to relax until we are utterly senseless, or climb Kilimanjaro, or tour every single wine cellar in France. When did it stop being okay to just spend a few days off puttering about? Of course the vacation can only start when we actually get there. In case you need reminding, *no one* gets off a long haul flight looking fabulous, but here are a few tips that can ease the pain.

HOW TO PACK

When you have a very quick trip where you have to put on a dress or a suit for a meeting, fold it around bubble wrap—the air in it, unlike tissue, moves with the garment, so it doesn't crease.

—*JoMalone*

Roll your clothes instead of folding—it reduces the amount of space taken up!

—*tibbytoos*

Store the cloth bags that new shoes come in in your suitcase to aid fast packing. When the time comes, I stuff them with under-wear, bikinis, socks and vests. Makes for fast, organized unpacking on arrival, too, and they double up inside beach bags to protect iPods, cameras, etc. Or use them to take laundry home in.

—*LauraBailey*

HOW TO PACK SHOES

Pack your shoes inside socks and your socks inside shoes.

—*Johanna*

HOW TO CLOSE A FULL SUITCASE

Can't zip up an overfull suitcase? Leave it overnight. The contents magically seem to sink.

—*Olwen*

HOW TO COPE WITH LOST LUGGAGE

If you are traveling with someone else, put half of your stuff in their case and half of theirs in yours; if one case does go missing, then you will have some stuff with you until the missing one turns up. Don't put anything with your full home address on the outside of the case, though.

—*COLIYTYHE*

Don't forget to make a list of all the items packed—you can even photograph them if they are laid out on your bed. This is helpful for insurance claims. Also have an accurate description of your suitcase dimensions, make, color, etc.

—*stephh*

HOW TO GET THE WRINKLES AND CREASES OUT OF YOUR CLOTHES

If you arrive at a hotel to find your shirt or dress wrinkled, hang it in the bathroom while you shower. Be sure to close the door and get the bathroom quite warm, damp, and steamy . . . the wrinkles disappear.

—*Melody*

HOW TO STOP LUGGAGE FROM SMELLING MUSTY

Keep old slivers of scented soap in the pockets.

—*Bianca*

A couple of drops of essential oil on a tissue in the pockets will keep luggage smelling sweet and also prevent bacteria and other nasties.

—*meeze*

Put a dryer sheet inside. This keeps the luggage from smelling musty while it's not being used. *And* a fresh dryer sheet included while packing for a trip will ensure that your clothes don't end up with that "cargo hold" smell upon arrival.

—*dabasan*

HOW TO ENSURE THAT LOSING YOUR PASSPORT DOESN'T RUIN YOUR VACATION

When traveling, keep a paper copy of your passport—if you lose your passport or if it's stolen, the copy will assist you to get a new one quickly.

—*Midge*

Scan your passport and e-mail it to yourself. If anything happens to it, just open your e-mail and print a copy.

—*IrishGirl*

HOW TO PROTECT AGAINST SPILLS WHILE TRAVELING

Always travel with resealable plastic bags. I pack everything inside them when traveling. You'll know why if you have ever had an accident with makeup or exploding shampoo. (You can also use them to make everything from marinated chicken to a body scrub with honey, salt, and lime oil.)

—*JoMalone*

HOW TO MAKE A LONG FLIGHT BEARABLE WITH AND FOR A THREE-YEAR-OLD WHO DOESN'T LIKE WATCHING FILMS

Try making a "vacation backpack," kind of like the ones you get from the airport for young children, and fill it with things like small toys (don't have to be expensive), a coloring book, and some special vacation crayons, etc.

It's all about the hype. Tell them that because they have been so good you've got a special treat for them to play with on the plane. That way they'll be really excited and just tuck straight into all the little games, etc. When I used to babysit, I'd go onto the Internet the night before and print loads of different coloring-in pages and small easy puzzles, staple them together, and make a glitzy customized front cover. Free fun!

 —sophie08

HOW TO REMOVE TAR PICKED UP
AT THE BEACH FROM YOUR FEET

Nail-polish remover works really well and so does baby oil or lighter fluid, believe it or not.

 —jsa

My grandmother always used butter. It works.

 —Leggbarbara

HOW TO KEEP MOSQUITOES AWAY

Take vitamin B supplements. It works really well.

 —Hobbit

Use tea tree oil. It's quite an earthy smell and you do get used to it, but insects hate it, particularly mosquitoes. A few dabs on vulnerable areas does the trick. I also rub it around window and door frames during the summer. The aroma keeps insects away.

 —carolec

· SAFETY ·

OR AS ONE PROPHET SAID, "BELIEVE IN GOD, BUT TETHER YOUR CAMEL."

ONCE you accept that there just are baddies out there who want to do us harm, the only possible response is, "Bummer. Now, what can I do to minimize my risk?" Safety issues are often a series of small precautions you can put in place, and which soon become habit. Once they are habit, you can forget about them. There is a lot to be said for vigilance, but if we allow our safety to preoccupy us, then we become paranoid. And two types of people, the totally reckless and the cripplingly paranoid, are equally boring to be around. Be sensible, be aware, and keep things in proportion.

HOW TO NOT BE TOTALLY STRANDED

When walking to your car, carry your car keys in one coat pocket and your cell phone in the other. That way, if your handbag is snatched, you can still call the police and get home.

—aspi80

HOW TO STAY SAFE DURING A STORM

When you find a storm is coming, head to the lower levels of your home. Try to get away from windows or glass. If you don't have a lower level, get to a door frame, or a closet as far away from the exterior walls of your house as possible. Having a wind-up or battery-powered radio will help to let you know when it is safe to move about your house again.

—ramee151

HOW TO WALK DOWN A DESERTED STREET OR ALLEY SAFELY AT NIGHT

What I do is carry my keys with each sticking out between my fingers. I also do a fake wave as though someone is waiting for me or has spotted me. I figure that I am less likely to be mugged if it looks like someone has seen me.

—nijago

1. Do not talk on your phone or listen to music. This will encourage attackers since it is obvious that you're distracted (the person on the end of the phone will not be able to do anything quickly enough, anyway).

2. Look around and behind you continuously as you walk.

3. Do not have your hood up and do keep your hair tucked in (women with short hair are less likely to be attacked than those with long hair).

4. Carry a rape alarm and have your thumb on the button as you walk.

5. If you do get attacked, shout "Help" repeatedly as loudly as possible and fight back; the attacker will be more likely to give up.

   —kate1989

I heard that it's better to shout "Fire" instead of "Help" because more people are likely to respond to something that could affect themselves—as horrible as it may sound.

—missmia

There is a legendary move that will at least delay an attacker. It's called a Schoolgirl; basically you kick the attacker in the shins and run. Sounds stupid, but it could work.

—Pixielixiefixie

Long hair can be used to grab you or hold on to you, and a ponytail is even worse. Tuck your hair into your collar. Walk tall, be aware, and don't be worried about offending someone who makes you nervous. Your instincts are the result of thousands of years of other human beings' experience; listen to them.

—Tatchull

HOW TO GUARD YOUR HANDBAG
IN A PUBLIC RESTROOM

Wash your hands in the basin nearest the hand dryer, or equip yourself with paper towels before washing, so that your handbag isn't left unguarded while you dry your hands.

—Cali

While in the stall, don't use the hook on the door to hang your purse; someone could grab it over the door and you'll be totally helpless. And who wants to put a purse on the bathroom floor? Put the strap around your neck!

—*LaterTater*

HOW TO DETER HOTEL THIEVES

If your hotel's security could be better, then always leave the DO NOT DISTURB sign hanging on your door. The maid may not come in to clean, but at least your possessions will be safe.

—*Samantha*

Make sure you leave the TV on (loud enough to be heard by anyone standing outside the hotel room door) before you leave your room. That should fool the thieves into thinking that someone's still in the room. If your hotel has an auto power-off mechanism activated when you take your key card off the card dock, ask for an extra key card from the front desk. (Hotels issue two key cards per room as standard, anyway.) That way you can carry one key card with you and leave the other one on the key dock to leave the power on for the TV.

—*rachney*

We never take any valuables with us and always, always use the safety deposit boxes for cash, passports, etc. The first thing we do on arrival is book one of those.

—*anassa*

HOW TO COPE WITH A HOTEL FIRE

Always check out the fire exit when you check in and always have a flashlight in your room. You might have to run down a pitch-dark staircase.

—*Melody*

HOW TO BE IDENTIFIED IN AN EMERGENCY

Make sure you have two numbers stored under the name "ICE" (In Case of Emergency) in your cell phone.

—*Flavia*

HOW TO ESCAPE A PLANE IN THE EVENT OF A CRASH

Make a note of how many seats there are between your seat and the emergency exit in front of (and behind) you. If the worst happens, it may be dark/smoky, so this way you can "count" your way to the nearest exit.

—*monkeyface*

HOW TO SURVIVE A FIRE

The most important thing, especially if you have children, is to have a fire drill and practice it. That way everyone is less likely to panic. Try to figure out as many ways as possible out of each room and prearrange a specific meeting place outside the house.

—*Tracy*

The fire department will come around to your house and advise on fire safety for free. Buy a fire blanket and an extinguisher, and test smoke alarms regularly.

—*Alexa*

HOW TO AVOID A FIRE CAUSED
BY FRYING FOOD IN HOT OIL

If your oil is getting too hot, turn down the heat and add more oil; the cold oil will immediately bring down the temperature. Emergency averted.

—*beagirl2*

You can tell when oil has reached a perfect frying temperature by inserting a wooden spoon as soon as it starts to get hot (make sure it's a *wooden* spoon; plastic may melt, and metal conducts heat), then turning the spoon so that its back is facing upward. When you first see tiny bubbles rising off the back of the spoon, your oil is hot enough to fry, but not hot enough to flash.

—*pcwallace*

1. If the oil starts to smoke, take the pan off the heat.

2. Oil will not simmer unless there is something in it, so don't wait for it to start simmering, no matter what the recipe tells you, because it won't; it'll burst into flames.

3. If the oil has started smoking, do not put the lid on the pan. It'll just burst into flames and the hot lid will go flying off and hit something.

Unfortunately these three fantastic tricks had to be learned the hard way.

—*wonder1woman*

HOW TO FIND A LOST CHILD WHILE OUT

We always tell our six-year-old son that if he gets separated from us while out to look for someone in a uniform (even in a shop, staff often can be identified) or a lady who looks like a granny. We have taught him our address and phone number, and he will sometimes wear a wristband with our cell phone numbers on it. We have also told him that if someone tries to take him away, he should shout "No, no, no; you're not my mom!" and make a fuss so he can draw attention to himself.

—*COLIYTYHE*

Write your cell phone number on the inside of their shirt/coat, and ask them to tell an adult to phone you if they get lost.

—*Gwiddon*

HOW TO LIST YOUR POSSESSIONS FOR INSURANCE

It's much easier to go around the house videotaping everything you own (with your own running commentary for details) than to write a huge list of all your possessions for insurance purposes. Just keep the video at your office, so that if everything does go up in smoke, the video won't go, too.

—*Olga*

HOW TO KEEP KEYS AND MONEY SAFE

Get an empty mayonnaise jar, paint it white inside, and store all your keys and money in there. No burglar would ever suspect it.

—*wnknt*

HOW TO DETER BURGLARS

If you have a driveway and you are away in your car on vacation, ask neighbors if they would park one of their cars in your driveway while you are not there.

—*COLIYTYHE*

HOW TO SCARE OFF INTRUDERS

If you're returning home and are scared that there might be someone inside your house, ring your own doorbell and leave plenty of time before you let yourself in. It should scare them off.

—*Enola*

HOW TO AVOID EYE INJURIES

Always strike matches away from you. A flying ember in the eye is not fun.

—*Rain*

HOW TO BE SAFE ON DATES

Watch for inconsistent behavior and for the bondage grip, when someone grabs your wrist in a way that throws you off balance.

Don't give out too much information about yourself in the first six dates.

Let your best friend know when you are going on a first date and have her call you—just in case you want to ditch him. And even if you think he's a keeper, call your BF when you go to the ladies' room and let her know where you are.

—*Masi*

HOW TO COPE WITH A VIOLENT PARTNER

No one should ever have to "cope" with a violent partner. If someone mistreats you, it means that he has no respect for you, and what is a relationship without respect?

The next time your partner gets violent, just leave. Don't try to fight back or reason. When people see red, they just see red. When he starts to become aggressive, just try to stay calm and leave the building. Go and stay with friends or family. Wait until the morning to speak to him. Tell him that his behavior is unacceptable. You deserve better. Get out before he gets out of control. Find someone else who will love and respect you and never think of hurting you.

—*sophie08*

Get help; you can't do it alone. It's not as simple as just telling him, "If you can make a fist, you can wrap your hand around the doorknob and get out." If you don't have a network of friends whom you can trust to help you (one friend alone can't do it and some well-meaning people make things worse), surf the net for a support group or a therapist who can lead you to a "safe house." Get yourself to the point where you decide that if you leave, you won't go back. And don't expect your partner to change.

—*Masi*

· GROWING OLDER ·
OR WHAT WAS I GOING TO SAY?

UNLESS you have the money to live in your own personal theme park, it is a very good idea to keep up. Keep up with music, fashion, news, and particularly technology. Each new device we get initially seems baffling, but spend an hour with the instruction manual and use it for a couple of days, and it is quickly second nature. Problems arise when we opt out, stating that we're technophobes and flatly refusing to engage. Very quickly the rest of the world overtakes us and we find ourselves increasingly out of step and irritated by modern life, as if we no longer speak the language. Keeping up, by taking each tiny step as it comes along, avoids a huge, uncomfortable leap later. The world changes, so you need to change with it, or else you'll find yourself isolated—which is scary—and annoyed.

HOW TO GROW OLD GRACEFULLY

Grow old disgracefully; it's more fun.

—*BamBam*

A playful child still resides in all of us, no matter your age. Let her out occasionally.

—*Snagglepusstoo*

HOW TO JOG YOUR MEMORY

If you can't remember why you crossed the room or went upstairs, retrace your steps exactly. The action might trigger your memory —if not, don't fret about it. Do something else.

—*Cali*

Tie a knot in your handkerchief. Next time you use your handkerchief, you'll be reminded of whatever it was. Then don't forget where you've put it.

—*catinthehat*

If I wake during the night and remember something important, I turn the clock away from the bed. In the morning I wonder why I've done that and usually remember. Or throw a pillow on the floor. Anything to jog your memory in the morning.

—*patsharp*

HOW TO REDUCE MUSCLE CRAMPS IN THE NIGHT

To avoid attacks of muscle cramp, drink one tumbler of tonic water (not low-cal) per day. This should give your system enough quinine to do the trick.

—*Cali*

HOW TO KEEP YOUR MIND SHARP

1. Play solitaire.
2. Stay positive.
3. Do crosswords.
4. Sing.
5. Smile, smile, smile.

   —*Redlady*

HOW TO IMPROVE YOUR MEMORY AND CONVERSATION SKILLS

Read something interesting (something as small as a news article or an Internet blog or even a tip you read here) and share it with a friend. Not only will you have read, but you'll probably have a great conversation, too.

   —*stelladore*

HOW TO AGE WELL

You age well by living well. This means taking care of yourself, but more important, being happy, learning from your mistakes and not making a big deal out of them.

There is nothing that looks better on an "aging" woman than happiness and a savoir faire that is attained only by living. Living is messy and full of mistakes. Living well means that we deal with these messy problems with grace, and this also shows in your face. Make no mistake: sunscreens, moisturizers, water, diet, and exercise are important; however, none of this will make an "aging" woman more appealing than having lived a full life and come out the other side happy!

   —*Byronspsbatt*

All things in moderation, and never hold a grudge, as it makes you bitter. Not good for wrinkle-free skin.

  —munchkin

Moisturize, moisturize, moisturize, and remember that your face doesn't end in the line on your chin where it slopes to become your neck. The décolletage is a very important area to moisturize since it is that area that becomes prominently aged in women's advanced years, specifically because of lack of moisture. I also find that the hands betray a woman's age, no matter how much aid her face has had, surgically or not. Having said all that, I think that part of the benefit of getting older is that we become more comfortable in our own skin, so if we enrich ourselves through knowledge and experience, then we add more value to ourselves as we grow older.

  —VerucaS

Remember, even when you have a pain, you don't have to be one.

  —Hetti

Growing old is inevitable; growing up is optional. *Don't* grow up!

  —Fayehf

HOW TO AGE HAPPILY

There is a saying: Life should not be a journey to the grave with the intention of arriving safely in an attractive and well-preserved body, but rather to skid in sideways, chocolate in hand, totally worn out, and screaming "WOO-HOO, what a ride!"

  —clinic2316

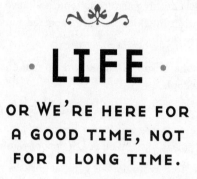

· LIFE ·

OR WE'RE HERE FOR A GOOD TIME, NOT FOR A LONG TIME.

HERE are the little recipes that make life smoother for you and for the people around you. This is the icing on the cake. Thank you for reading this book; if you remember even half of the tips in it, you'll be considered a genius.

HOW TO BLUFF

When you know nothing about the topic and have been engaged in a conversation in which you are expected to contribute, try the following:

1. Crack a joke. If you can make one up fast enough, this can distract people.

2. Ask the other person questions. People love to blather on.

3. Steer the conversation into a different arena: "But didn't you find it was . . . ," "Well yes, it sort of reminds me of . . ."

4. Be vague. Toss around a few general phrases.

5. Violently agree with the other person's opinion, thus prompting them to share views you can then pass off as your own.

6. Excuse yourself from the situation. Ask them to hold that thought; you're just going for a refill. Pretend you felt your phone vibrating. Anything.

   —buddha

HOW TO WIN AN ARGUMENT

Figure out the other person's point of view and ask questions— people are more likely to change their mind if they feel they are being heard. And flatter relentlessly—but not obviously.

   —Tawny

If you want to win, act calm and bemused about the whole situation; this will really work them into a rage while you look calm and collected. Then shrug, smile, and walk away and leave them fuming and looking like a twit.

   —Khlovechild14

HOW TO RESPOND TO A RUDE QUESTION

"I'll forgive you for asking if you'll forgive me for not answering."
Short, sweet, devastatingly simple.

   —*CeeVee*

Answer with a question. "Why would you want to know that?" or
"What sort of a question is that?" works quite well—put the dis-
comfort back onto the person asking the rude question.

   —*Allflagsflying*

One simple word response: *"Why?"* That should be enough to
shift the pressure onto the asker . . . and don't let them get away
with answering "Because I want to know." Press on with, "Why?"

   —*Julia Farber*

Answer a rude question with complete silence. Just look at the
person with a blank expression and say nothing. When they ask
why you don't answer, say, "I just can't believe you asked that."
Works every time.

   —*asildem*

HOW TO NOT GET NERVOUS AT PARTIES

Get there early-ish; it's easier to meet people when there are only
a few other guests.

   —*Nerissa*

Surrounded by strangers? Imagine each is as ill-at-ease as you
are and decide to make each person you talk to comfortable. If it
doesn't work with one person, move on to the next. The idea is to
focus on the other person and not on yourself.

   —*asildem*

Wiggle. Just a little wiggle, be it at your desk, in your kitchen, or on the street . . . shake that beautiful butt and I bet you'll smile. You can wiggle a little or a lot, in private or with the world (just know that others may stare).

    —ajbird

Before you go to sleep, write five good feelings you have had today.

    —peplow

Always remember . . . we're here for a good time, not for a long time! Live every day as though it's your last, live with no regrets, try to be positive about every situation because somehow negativity has a way of reflecting itself on your entire life, career, family, friends, etc. . . .

    —123karla123

A schoolteacher taught me this, and after eleven years, I still remember it. Happiness comes from having:

1. Something to do

2. Someone to love

3. Something to look forward to.

    —Angelina

If it doesn't enhance your life, *get rid of it.*

    This works particularly well with guys; I've got rid of two with this advice and I'm happy!

    —danni01

I find it helpful to remember that I am one lucky SOB to have been born in a country of power and money where women are allowed to be individuals. That I have so much potential and so many open doors in my life, and if I sit here wasting it, thinking about how I wish my thighs were smaller, then I am pathetic for doing nothing of substance with all that I have. And a good run never hurts, either.

—rsjdooley

You can have only one thought in your head at a time, so make it a positive one.

—karenannerichards

HOW TO SPOT A PHONEY

We are what we actually do, not what we say.

—Greer

HOW NOT TO BE SAD DURING THOSE DARK WINTER MONTHS

This is a simple solution that helps me. I live alone, so in the winter I leave my apartment in the dark and get home in the dark. I plugged a lamp into a timer and set it so it turned on a few minutes before I got back from work. It makes home feel more welcoming and is great to have a little light when struggling with keys and whatever else I am carrying.

—Melaniezelanie

HOW TO LOVE YOURSELF

"Fake it till you make it!" If you cannot think of good things about yourself, are depressed, etc., then fake feeling good about yourself until you realize how worthy you are of loving yourself. This is a tactic that works very well in many instances and situations. Since you are responsible for your own happiness and behavior, it is your responsibility to fake having a good time until you actually relax and begin having a good time. This does not make you a shallow person. On the contrary, this makes you a smart person who takes her own destiny into her own hands. Take control of your life and emotions today!

—*Byronspsbatt*

HOW TO RECOVER (SOCIALLY) AFTER A NIGHT OF DRINKING TOO MUCH AND EMBARRASSING YOURSELF

When you make an ass of yourself, it is always better to laugh at yourself than to be embarrassed. Follow up by retelling the story (poetic license allowed) to friends over cocktails.

—*rachbu*

Remember that unless you were turning pantyless cartwheels halfway through a formal dinner party, everyone else is, as always, thinking about what they did and not about what you did.

—*lemes*

HOW TO ADJUST AFTER A MOVE TO A NEW TOWN

E-mail all your friends and tell them to give you any contacts in the new place. Then be brave and cold call. Give *everyone* a chance, however weird they sound on the phone or e-mail. Or hold a party for all the people whose names you were given.

—*LevantineLass*

HOW TO GET PEOPLE TO LISTEN TO YOU

Never apologize, unless something very important has gone very wrong and someone's feelings are actually hurt. Stop apologizing before you speak, apologizing for being in the way, apologizing for interrupting, apologizing for taking up space. You don't see men apologizing every five minutes, do you? And they don't get mad at each other or dislike each other for it—in fact, they don't even notice.

—*scoop*

HOW TO STOP BEING SUCH A CHATTERBOX

Someone asked me something once that really struck a chord with me: "Are you listening, or are you waiting to talk?" This changed the way I participated in conversations. I do not want to be someone who is sitting in a conversation just waiting for my turn to talk. You learn so much by listening, but if you are doing the talking, in most cases you don't learn something new. I know it's hard when you're nervous, but perhaps try taking a deep breath and reminding yourself of those things: If I listen instead of talking, I will learn something that I may not have known before. Ask open-ended questions of the people you are with. That will allow them to do the talking.

—*kate42*

HOW TO SILENCE YOUR INNER CRITIC

What I do is yell at the inner critic and tell it to shut the hell up. Seriously. When you find yourself putting yourself down, be your own best friend and defend yourself. I find that some of the things I consider my largest, most terrible faults are either unrecognizable to others or they find them endearing.

—*Rnotghi*

HOW TO STOP BEING LATE AND RUSHED ALL THE TIME

I am chronically late, but recently I made two changes that seem to help:

Add fifteen minutes to the amount of time you think it will take to get somewhere. I never anticipate how long it will take me to actually get out the door; e.g., if I know it takes me thirty minutes to get somewhere, I usually leave exactly thirty minutes to get there. What I don't realize is that it takes fifteen minutes to find my keys, get my cell phone, etc.

Don't set appointments you know you can't meet. I tend to say "Sure, I can be there by five," even if I *know* I will have to race around. Now I try to be more reasonable. If I say, "You know what, I'm going to need until five thirty," then I actually show up a bit early. Everyone is happy!

—*Angelina*

HOW TO COPE WITH EMPTY-NEST SYNDROME WHEN YOUR YOUNGEST HAS LEFT HOME AND YOUR HUSBAND DOESN'T UNDERSTAND WHY YOU'RE SO SAD

The answer is to *get busy*! (It will take your mind off it if nothing else.) Find something you love doing, whether it's taking a course or even fund-raising for a charity. It might help you remember who you were before you were a mother.

—*Ulrika*

HOW TO SUPPORT A BEREAVED FRIEND

I write at the time of the death, but I also put a note in my diary, six months ahead, to prompt me to write a follow-up note or touch base with a phone call then. Often people think that six months down the line, life is back to normal and that the worst of the grieving is over. But it really isn't. Someone did this for me when my sister died—and I have made a point of doing the same ever since.

—*Carok*

Please remember when phoning to listen and not use the bereaved to listen to your own story. My friend whose mother died two weeks ago said that everyone she spoke to had a dead-mother story to tell her and tried to compete with everything she wanted to say.

—*Loladoc*

HOW TO WRITE A CONDOLENCE/SYMPATHY LETTER

Many people never get around to writing sympathy notes because, as they say, "I just don't know what to say." Turns out, that's exactly the *right* thing to say. Just write a brief sentence or two: "Dear So-and-So, I heard about your loss and I just don't know what to say. I'm thinking of you." Short and sweet, and far better than doing nothing at all.

—*CeeVee*

I always put, "Please don't reply, but I'll call you in a few weeks," which makes me call and speak to them.

—*pam*

HOW TO COPE WITH BEREAVEMENT

Allow yourself time to grieve. Seriously. Sounds simple, but it's imperative. Give in to whatever it is you are feeling and let go. If you need to sob, find a quiet place and let 'er rip. If you want to laugh, do it! And, don't feel guilty about it, either. Nearly every emotion you have is justified and warranted. It takes time. How much? Well, that depends. Take the time that you need and don't feel guilty about it.

—*Emmar*

My advice is to talk about the people you have lost, share all the good times, but most of all cherish the living. Talk to them, enjoy them, take pictures of them, record them on video, and make voice tapes; all these things will remind you, when they pass, of how lucky you were to have known them.

—*jeanharte*

One day at a time! Watch out for anniversaries such as the deceased's birthday; they creep up on you and can be tough to get through. We usually plan to do something as a family on my son's birthday. It's as if we are marking the day but keeping busy and distracted, too. If you've lost someone through illness (maybe cancer), then try using your grief as an energy source and do some fund-raising. I found that quite therapeutic.

Let your family and friends help, too; they're probably not sure how to handle the situation, either.

Give yourself time—lots of it; there's no right or wrong way to cope, you just have to.

—COLIYTYHE

HOW TO GET REVENGE

Don't let those people have one more minute of your soul! Living well is the best revenge, and while you go about living well, working hard, and doing for others, you will gradually heal yourself from the hurt that was imposed on you. Take the high road; it leads to much nicer places.

—asildem

A subtle but effective revenge tactic: batteries. Turn every battery from every appliance in the house the wrong way around. Do not remove them! If they've been removed, then it becomes obvious what's happened. You want him to wonder if all his stuff is broken. That means the TV remote, mouse, keyboard, power tools, anything! It'll drive him mad for weeks.

—AnnaLehane

HOW TO ACCEPT A COMPLIMENT

A warm thank-you and a smile is all that's required. It seems dead obvious, but it took me forever to realize. I used to babble about where I got said dress, etc. out of surprise or even embarrassment. The truth is, if the complimenter wants to know, he or she will ask a follow-up question.

   —*janicody*

HOW TO GAIN CONFIDENCE

When I am feeling a bit incompetent and need a boost, I simply lift my chin. It straightens out my back, I stand taller, and people look in my face, not at my forehead.

   —*Erin helgren*

Remember that dreaming of the person you'd like to be is wasting the person you are!

   —*Louie*

Act the part. You'll eventually feel confident with time. Remember, no one knows how you truly feel inside. Before any big presentations or meetings, I remind myself that no one knows I'm nervous and they won't know if I've made a mistake unless I tell them. Just like performers—they mess up all the time, but the audience never knows!

   —*mikookie*

HOW TO STOP BEING BITCHY

Bitching reflects worse on the person who is doing the bitching than on the victims themselves, so if you find yourself making an unnecessary nasty comment about somebody who has actually done you no wrong, then work out why it is you're actually doing it. . . . You'll often find that it's because secretly you are jealous of them in some way, in which case, it's really not their fault or their problem, but rather it's your own.

—*Urmila*

HOW TO MAKE YOURSELF MORE ATTRACTIVE

Get rid of your emotional baggage . . . anger, resentment, and worry all show up in your looks, so battle your demons and let go of issues that are in the past or out of your control. Once you have done so, it will feel as though a huge weight has been lifted off your shoulders and you will positively glow from within. This is the best beauty advice I've been given and it works.

—*Urmila*

HOW TO SOUND GOOD ON THE PHONE

Smile when you talk on the phone. Even though the people on the other end can't see it, they can hear it in your voice.

—*Melissaann124*

You're a lot less likely to sound nervous on the phone if you talk while you're lying down on your back. It relaxes your throat muscles (which is also the reason why people snore when they lie down to sleep), so you don't sound at all shaky. I record my voice mail message like that, too, and it always sounds carefree and breezy.

—*hbkt83*

I find that standing up during a call makes me much more assertive—great when I am contacting utility services.

—*Redlady*

Especially when I'm nervous about a phone call, I will stand on a chair as I talk. Something about it makes me feel brave and disconnected from my nervousness. Also, I imagine the surprise on the face of the person I am speaking with if they could see me ... priceless!

—*flytink*

HOW TO COMMENT ON A BOOK HIGHLY RECOMMENDED BY A FRIEND THAT YOU'VE FOUND CHILDISH AND BORING

Tell your friend the book was "incredible." You don't have to add incredibly childish and incredibly boring.

—*Catinthehat*

HOW TO KNOW WHICH LINE TO CHOOSE WHEN THERE'S MORE THAN ONE

Always choose the line to the left. Apparently, most people's natural tendency is to go to the right.

—*sandrasimmons*

HOW TO FIGURE OUT WHETHER YOU'RE FLUENT IN ANOTHER LANGUAGE

My Spanish professor at the University of Texas told me that when you dream in another language, you are fluent.

—*sandrasimmons*

HOW TO REMEMBER THINGS

When I'm away from home, I call myself and leave a message on my home answering machine. That way it can remain there until I complete the task.

—Majella716

HOW TO GET A SIGNAL ON YOUR CELL PHONE

If you have no signal and really need to send a text, put the phone on your head, which will boost the signal . . . it works!

—Channers89

HOW TO FIX A WET CELL PHONE

I accidentally dropped my cell phone down the toilet—I used the hair dryer and after around fifteen minutes, the phone was working perfectly.

—Redlady

I have ruined three cell phones due to "water damage." I recently washed my boyfriend's cell phone in the washing machine, and the lady at the cell phone store mentioned that we could try putting the cell phone in dry white rice. We had it in for two days and violà! The phone works! Saved me $250!

—sugarstar

HOW TO REMEMBER PASSWORDS

Find a word that will always be on your desk, for example, the make of your computer monitor (normally printed on the front of it). Even if you don't use this exact word and you add numbers/letters, it should jog your memory when you've forgotten.

—PaperCut

HOW TO LOOK GLAMOROUS IN A PHOTOGRAPH

Turn your body to a 45-degree angle to the camera, then turn your neck so that your face is toward the camera. Place one foot slightly in front of the other, with that leg bent slightly at the knee. Lift your chin just a little bit, and smile! If you're being posed with someone you dislike, or your hair/clothes/makeup are horrible, don't try to get out of it—just close your eyes. Most people won't keep, or pass on, those pictures.

—*Onesweettart*

Look down the lens of the camera as if you are looking at your lover and you want to make passionate love to him. Do this with a smile and you won't look like a porn star.

—*jennyp*

If the photographer counts one, two, three, smile on the count of two. Your smile will look more natural and less frozen or fake.

—*patriciao*

My daughter-in-law gave me some good advice: If you're not happy with your tummy area and you're having a photograph taken with your partner, put your arms around his waist and conceal a third of your body behind his—makes you look like a loving couple and hides the wobbly bits!

—*Blodwen*

HOW TO STOP CHOKING

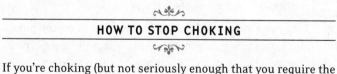

If you're choking (but not seriously enough that you require the Heimlich maneuver), the quickest way to regain your composure is to raise your arms above your head. It does something to your chest, lungs, or diaphragm—whatever, it works.

—*Gam*

HOW TO BE SEXY WITHOUT OVERDOING IT

"Sexy" is a state of mind, not a way of behaving. Be comfortable in your own skin—be yourself. *Smile*—men say that's sexy. Laugh. Don't be so concerned about what clothes you wear, how your hair looks, if your makeup is perfect. Some of the sexiest women in the world are not the most beautiful; they just come across that way because they exude confidence, playfulness, and humor.

—*Inmop*

HOW TO BE A GOOD GUEST

A postcard sent the next day is even better than a phone call. Always try to imagine that the hostess hasn't had a single thank-you and that she was just wondering whether anyone had had a good time that night. Something received through the post is always lovely.

—*LevantineLass*

HOW TO MAKE GUESTS COMFORTABLE

When having overnight guests:

1. Place a tray in the guest room with water bottles, something sweet, something savory, and a current magazine or book that would match their interests.

2. Turn down their bed at night and put a mint on the pillow. This costs practically nothing and you will be amazed at your guest's response. This is a good thing to let your children do. They learn how to care for others and get a ton of praise from the guest for doing it.

—*sandrasimmons*

HOW TO STOP GETTING BED SPINS
WHEN YOU'VE HAD A FEW DRINKS

If you lie down with one foot on the floor, it seems to "ground" you.

    —Curles2007

HOW TO KEEP AN INVASIVE
MOTHER-IN-LAW UNDER CONTROL

Mark in your diary one day of the week (e.g., Tuesdays at 8 p.m.) when *you* will call her for fifteen minutes. Listen, be nice, make small talk, and hang up after fifteen minutes ("Sorry, got to go; someone's at the door."). The rest of the week let the machine pick it up when she calls (get a phone with caller ID or a special ring for her number). She will eventually catch on and call less and, more important, she will have nothing to complain to your husband about. It sounds a bit radical, I know, but it's my mother's advice to me and it has worked for her for more than thirty years.

    —zica

HOW TO HANDLE PROSPECTIVE IN-LAWS

Never let them hear you saying anything but nice things about anyone ever. Make a practice of saying good things about people, and stick up for people. Help Mom in the kitchen and load the dishwasher—don't ask, "Can I help you?" Just do it quietly without making a thing of it, as if you were helping your own mother.

    —operatix

HOW TO STOP ARGUING WITH YOUR MOTHER

If the things you argue over are silly, then try not opposing her. While you are letting your mother win silly arguments, go about living your life with dignity and maturity. If the arguments are about things that are more serious, then make a point of showing her that you are considering her opinion. She does, after all, have a lifetime of experience. Acknowledge that, even if you choose not to follow her advice.

—*asildem*

Treat your mom like you would treat one of your friends. When she comes in, offer to make her a drink. If she is struggling with something, offer to help.

As she appreciates this, she will mellow toward you. Treat her like you would want to be treated and you'll find it should work.

It's all about respect and tolerance, not for your elders and betters and parents and children but for another human being. Of course I'm a mother answering this one; I have a twenty-two-year-old daughter. Yes, she drives me mad sometimes, but guess what? I do the same to her.

—*Sheepish239*

HOW TO HELP MAINTAIN A GOOD RELATIONSHIP WITH YOUR MOTHER

The more often you call her, the less time it will take. If you only speak once a month, she'll expect a worthwhile conversation; if you speak every day, five minutes will do. Conversely, the more often you talk to someone, the more there is to say.

—*Cali*

ACKNOWLEDGMENTS

With sincere thanks to:

Mum, Humphrey, Sarah, Alex, Aleese, and Dad (who was an infinite source of crap top tips); I love them all very much.

All my family and friends who were so generous with their support and top tips, particularly Annabel Rivkin and Catherine Heeschen for their wit, and Natalie Massenet, founder of net-a-porter.com, who taught me how to be a twenty-first-century girl.

Kate Lee and Karolina Sutton at ICM, who continue to answer my midnight, stream-of-consciousness e-mails.

Carrie Thornton at Three Rivers, who made this an infinitely better book.

Groovytrain, the company that designed and built toptipsforgirls.com.

And profound thanks to all the wise and generous women who contribute tips to the website and thus this book. In particular, the current top tipsters: COLIYTYHE, CeeVee, Sophie08, Masi, operatix, Redlady, LevantineLass, sandrasimmons, vaportrailed, and Cali.

INDEX

ABOUT THE AUTHOR

KATE REARDON has spent twenty years at the cutting edge of women's publishing. She started as a fashion assistant at *American Vogue* and at twenty-one was made fashion editor of *Tatler*. She has contributed to most major British newspapers and written three columns in the *Times*—which named her one of Britain's best writers. She is currently a contributing editor at *Vanity Fair*. She lives in London during the week and spends the weekends at her cottage in the Wiltshire countryside—as she works from home, she finds this helps her remember what day of the week it is.